DATE DUE	
3·1·95		
7-5-95		
OCT 2 8 2014		

Surgical Endodontics
Colour Manual

Surgical Endodontics
Colour Manual

I. E. Barnes, PhD, FDS RCS, BDS
Professor, Department of Operative Dentistry,
University of Newcastle upon Tyne Dental School

with contributions by

R. Palmer, PhD, FDS RCS, BDS
Senior Lecturer, Department of Periodontology,
UMDS, London

D. G. Smith, PhD, FDS RCS, DRD
Consultant, Department of Periodontology, Dental Hospital,
Newcastle upon Tyne

A. F. Carmichael, HDD, RFPS, FDS RCS, FDS RCPS
Senior Lecturer and Consultant, Conservation Department and
Department of Child Dental Health,
Glasgow Dental Hospital and School, Glasgow

Wright
London Boston Singapore Sydney Toronto Wellington

Wright
An imprint of Butterworth–Heinemann Ltd
Halley Court, Jordan Hill, Oxford OX2 8EJ

 PART OF REED INTERNATIONAL P.L.C.

OXFORD LONDON GUILDFORD BOSTON
MUNICH NEW DELHI SINGAPORE SYDNEY
TOKYO TORONTO WELLINGTON

First published by MTP Press Ltd 1984
Second imprint 1991

© **I.E. Barnes 1991**

British Library Cataloguing in Publication Data

Barnes, I. E. (Ian E) *1939–*
    Surgical endodontics.
    1. Dentistry. Endodontics. Surgery
I. Title   II. Palmer, R.   III. Smith, D. G.
    617.6342059

ISBN 0-7236-1571-3

Library of Congress Cataloging in Publication Data

    Data applied for

    0-7236-1571-3

peset by Scribe Design, Gillingham, Kent
in Scotland by Cambus Litho Ltd, Glasgow

Contents

Introduction

This book is derived from a series of articles written for dental practitioners and was first published in *Dental Update*. The articles were written as a consequence of running a weekly clinic, concerned largely with the correction of referred endodontic problems. In most cases the 'problems' did not exist and were treated simply by redoing the root filling or by undertaking a straightforward apicectomy. Regrettably, in many other cases, the problem would not have existed had the previously undertaken, and potentially simple, apicectomy been carried out competently.

There is no good reason why apical surgery should not be undertaken by the general dental practitioner as part of the patient's overall treatment. After all, the problem will usually have arisen either during, or as a result of, routine dental treatment. In addition, the tooth may require to be restored, either at the time of surgery or fairly soon thereafter. Regrettably, inexperience in the handling of soft tissues, and concern about the risk of damage to associated structures, often deters the dentist from attempting what is, if sensibly approached, an uncomplicated minor dento-alveolar operation.

Chapters 1–8 introduce the reader to the basic techniques of apicectomy. Chapters 9, 11, 12, 16 and 17 will, it is hoped, help the interested dentist to develop a competence to treat more complex cases, once he or she has become proficient in the basic skills.

The techniques described are those that I use, and experienced operators may well remark upon a number of omissions. My surgical prejudices are also evident, but I have taken the view that in a manual, as opposed to a textbook, a standpoint is of more value than a welter of opinion.

It is assumed that the reader has a competent working knowledge of important related subjects, such as pathology, medicine, pharmacology, anatomy and basic endodontics. If not, he or she must consult the appropriate expert texts.

It has been suggested that this book may also be of value in undergraduate training. I hope that this may be so, but would see it being of use only after the student has received a sound training in the theory and practice of simple dento-alveolar surgery.

The observant reader will remark upon the inadequate standard of conservation shown in a number of the illustrations. After treatment patients are referred to their dentist for the necessary restoration of the apicected tooth. On occasions such treatment had not been done by the time of the review appointment.

Preface to 2nd imprint

This is not a second edition. However, reprinting has allowed me to correct a few factual and textual errors that were present in the original book. Some concepts have been updated and two new sections added.

The first print was criticized by some, understandably perhaps, for not including references. However, the occasional selective reference is pretty weak beer, and those who wish for a detailed historical and 'academic' perspective may wish to read the chapter entitled 'Surgical Endodontics' in *Endodontics in Clinical Practice,* 3rd edition by F. J. Harty, published by Wright, 1990.

The original purpose of this manual remains; namely, to offer students and dentists a well illustrated practical guide to simple, reliable surgical endodontic technique.

Acknowledgements

Learning is a continuous process. Nevertheless, a basic philosophy is forged very early on by one's teachers; I am grateful to Mr D. Brock, Professor J. Moore, and Professor R. O'Neil, who taught me surgical technique, and the management of patients; and to Mr J. J. Messing, whose ingenuity and enthusiasm have advanced the practice of endodontics.

I have been greatly helped by many colleagues who have either photographed my work, or allowed me to photograph theirs. Such assistance has come from my House Surgeons over the past eight years, and, more specifically, from Esmond Corbett, Peter Floyd, David Gouk, Richard Palmer, Peter Rosenkranz, Ian Waite and Bill White, all of whom are, or have been, teachers at the Royal Dental Hospital School of Dental Surgery, London.

Mrs Betty Fisher has stoically retyped many drafts of the text, which has been expertly edited by Mr P. Johnstone.

Finally, the original articles on which this book is based would not have been written without encouragement and advice from the late Mrs Belle Maudsley, and from Miss Sue Kay, both of *Dental Update*.

To all these people, and to others I have not mentioned, my thanks are due.

I. E. Barnes
Corbridge, Northumberland
June 1984

Chapter 1

Principles of Apicectomy Technique

The term apicectomy is one that is commonly employed and will be used in this manual. However, the word is misleading because it places undue emphasis on a relatively trivial part of the surgical procedure.

A successful apicectomy technique depends partly on surgical skills, but as importantly on a logical approach, which must be based on a sound knowledge of endodontic theory.

The Apical Constriction

The principal aims when root filling are, first, to cleanse the root canal of debris and, second, to obturate it to the base of the apical constriction with some form of filling material so that noxious matter cannot escape into the supporting tissues.

The apical constriction is of the greatest importance to the success of endodontic therapy. It acts as a barrier to the passage of debris during instrumentation and as a stop for instruments, cement and the filling point. Following obturation of the root canal, the constriction becomes occluded with cementum which forms a physiological barrier (Figure 1.1). Once noxious matter has ceased to pass from the canal into the tissues surrounding the tooth, the body's defence and repair mechanisms will satisfactorily resolve the majority of apical lesions (Figure 1.2).

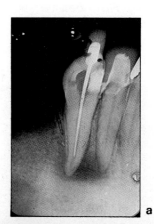

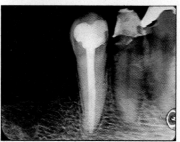

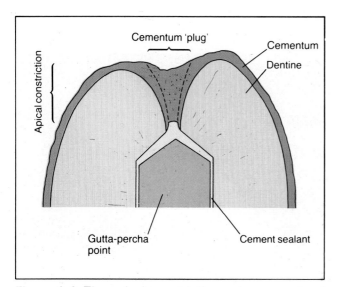

Figure 1.1 *The apical constriction acts as a natural 'stop' to the passage of instruments and debris. When the canal is properly filled the apical foramen will eventually become occluded with cementum*

Figure 1.2 a, b, *Repair of apical lesion following a conventional orthograde root-filling (review – 14 months)*

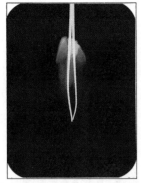

Figure 1.3 *Silver points passed down the buccal and lingual canals of a lower incisor. The cementation of either **one** of these points would probably have effected an apical seal. Removal of the root-tip during apicectomy will result in failure unless **both** canals are filled*

The apical constriction is also a valuable safeguard against the consequences of diagnostic error. For example, in the case of the lower incisor illustrated in Figure 1.3, the obturation of either the buccal or the lingual root canal would probably effect an adequate apical seal because both canals converge and join at the end of the root. Resection of the root-tip during apicectomy would result in eventual failure unless both canals had been identified and filled.

When a tooth is apicected, the apical constriction is removed with the terminal portion of root. As a result, the chances of long-term endodontic success are reduced for three reasons. First, because the root canal is exposed at a more coronal level, where it is larger in cross-section. A cemental barrier is less likely to form over this relatively large area of (non-physiological) root-filling material than it is within the small apical constriction (Figure 1.4). Second, because removal of the root-tip may expose a second, possibly unrecognized root canal (*see* Figure 1.3). Third, because some canals are so irregular in cross-section that they cannot be instrumented to a circular shape and thus the greater part of the apical seal may be comprised of cement sealant (Figure 1.5). Should the sealant be soluble, it may over the years be lost into the tissues, so that a dead-space develops between the filling-point and canal wall. If this occurs the filling may fail. The use of an insoluble cement may prevent such a loss, but in practice the problem is usually overcome by placing an insoluble sealant in the irregular terminal portion of the canal (Figure 1.6). Silver amalgam is most often used for this purpose and is termed a 'retrograde filling'. If the absence of signs and symptoms is used as a measure, amalgam can be considered to be well tolerated by the body. However, histological and radiological evidence suggests that amalgam may cause a mild foreign-body reaction in the adjacent tissues. There is, in addition, an increasing concern about levels of mercury absorption and toxicity. A retrograde amalgam filling must therefore be considered a poor substitute for the physiological seal that is formed by cementum within the apical constriction as the result of a successful root filling.

An 'apicectomy' should not be considered to be an elective procedure, but should be undertaken only when conventional orthograde root filling techniques are impracticable or have failed.

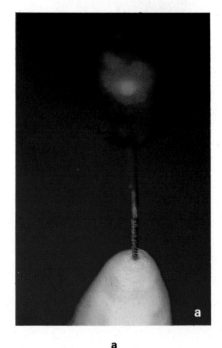

a

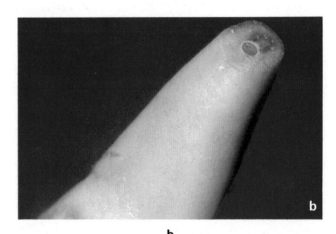

b

Figure 1.4 a, *The tip of a No. 15 file just fits into the apical foramen of this upper central incisor.* **b,** *The surface area of the gutta-percha and cement sealant that are exposed following removal of the root-tip is far greater than that of the intact apical foramen*

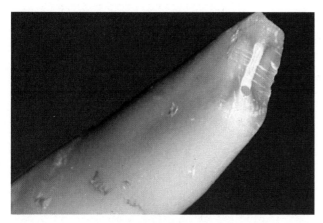

Figure 1.5 *It is not possible to instrument some canals to a circular shape. When such a canal is exposed following resection of the root apex, an excessive amount of soluble cement lute will lie in contact with the tissues*

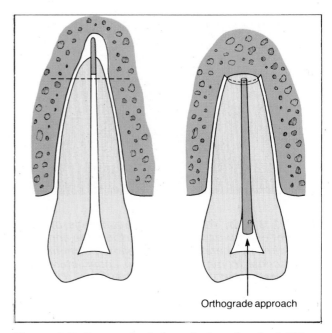

Orthograde approach

Figure 1.7 *Removal of the misplaced apical filling, and resection of the root-tip, allows the root canal to be instrumented and sealed by way of an orthograde approach*

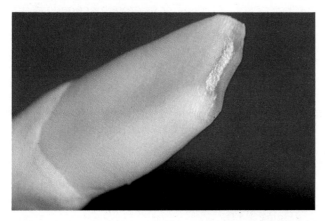

Figure 1.6 *The terminal 3 mm of the root canal, seen in Figure 1.5, has been run out with a bur and sealed by the placement of an insoluble retrograde amalgam filling*

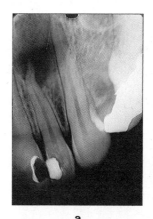 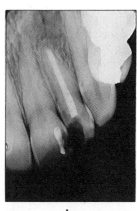

a   b

Figure 1.8 a, b, *Apicectomy and curettage of cyst. The root canal was obturated with gutta-percha and Tubliseal, placed by way of the orthograde approach at the time of operation (review – 1 year)*

Apicectomy Techniques

There are three basic apicectomy techniques and these must be clearly distingushed:

(1) Orthograde seal
(2) Orthograde + Retrograde seal
(3) Retrograde seal

Orthograde seal

This technique is used where surgical removal of the apical segment of root allows the rest of the root canal to be fully instrumented and properly filled by way of the crown; for example, when treating endodontic failure caused by an overextended sectional silver point (Figure 1.7), when a root-tip is abnormally bent, or when an apical lesion is to be investigated (Figure 1.8).

Orthograde + Retrograde seal

If the apical part of the root canal is irregular in cross-section it may be necessary to reinforce the apical seal by placing a retrograde amalgam in addition to obturating the canal with a cemented point or points (Figures 1.6 and 1.9).

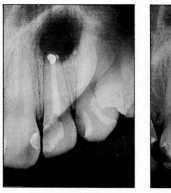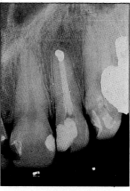

<table>
<tr><td align="center">a</td><td align="center">b</td></tr>
</table>

Figure 1.9 a, b, *Apicetomy and curettage of cyst. The root canal was filled by the orthograde approach at the time of operation but the narrow terminal part of the canal (commonly found in upper lateral incisors) was sealed with amalgam (review – 1 year)*

Retrograde seal

A simple retrograde seal is placed as a last resort when the coronal parts of the root canal are inaccessible, or impassable, with the consequence that a conventional root canal filling cannot be placed (Figure 1.10).

Long-term failure is slightly more likely when this technique is used, for the following reasons (Figure 1.11).

(1) Some part of the canal may remain uncleansed and unfilled with the risk that noxious matter may pass into the periodontal tissues by way of lateral canals.

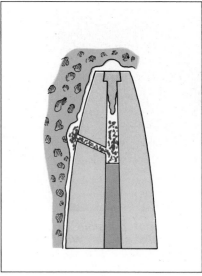

Figure 1.11 *The disadvantages of the simple retrograde seal are: (a) inability to properly condense the amalgam, (b) the possibility of overfilling the canal, thus preventing future post preparation and (c) the risk that noxious matter may pass into the tissues via lateral canals*

(2) If the canal is wide it may not be possible to condense the amalgam adequately, thus allowing the passage of toxins into the supporting tissues as the result of marginal leakage.

(3) Overfilling of the canal with amalgam may prevent the subsequent placement or replacement of a post (Figure 1.12).

Great improvements have been made in endodontic instrumentation over recent years. Curved or narrow canals that might previously have had to be dealt with by apicectomy techniques can now be treated conventionally. Surgical intervention is increasingly a matter

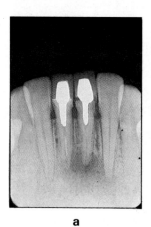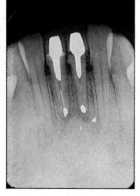

<table>
<tr><td align="center">a</td><td align="center">b</td></tr>
</table>

Figure 1.10 a, *Apicectomy $\overline{1|1}$ and curettage of apical lesion. $\overline{|2}$ was vital. Because of the gold posts retrograde seals alone were placed.* **b,** *Review – 1 year. Apical bone reformation is incomplete, although the teeth were asymptomatic. There is a loss of supporting bone, related to the poor crown margins, for the correction of which the patient had been referred to her general dental practitioner*

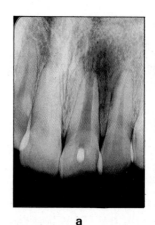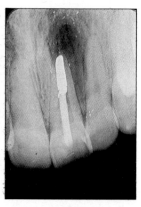

<table>
<tr><td align="center">a</td><td align="center">b</td></tr>
</table>

Figure 1.12 a, b, *Apicectomy and curettage of apical lesion. Despite the use of a large gutta-percha point to act as a 'stop', the retrograde amalgam fills too much of the canal (review – 11 months). See comments on the immature apex on page 16*

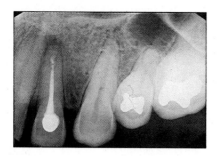

Figure 1.13 *Simple failure. No apical seal was placed in ⌊2 at operation 2 years previously*

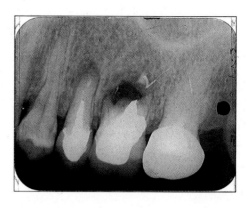

Figure 1.14 *Resounding failure. All three roots ⌊6 were apicected in theatre. The tip of one root remains. No apical seals were placed. There is a buccopalatal communication. The patient had been referred for the treatment of ⌊5! (Radiograph kindly sent to author. Reported case)*

of last resort, and usually requires a retrograde seal to be placed. Thus, the least effective surgical technique most often has to be used, putting a premium upon careful planning and meticulous technique.

A depressingly high number of failed apicectomies are referred for further treatment; and frequently examination shows that, although the apex of the root has been resected, there has been no attempt to create an apical seal. Such an approach displays either an astounding ignorance, or a total disregard, of basic theory. Figures 1.13 and 1.14 illustrate two such cases.

Chapter 2

Indications for Apicectomy

The principal indications for apicectomy are listed below, subdivided according to the operative technique that is usually best used.

When the Root Canal can be Instrumented and Fully Filled by a Coronal Approach following Removal of the Apical Segment (Orthograde or Orthograde + Retrograde)

(1) Failed root fillings that can be removed from the canal:

Apicectomy is sometimes indicated in the case of overextended root fillings because the apical constriction has been destroyed by instrumentation and a good seal cannot thereafter be achieved by conventional methods. A failure resulting from *underfilling* should be corrected in the first instance by refilling to the correct length and not by surgical means.

Root fillings may appear on radiographs to be properly placed at the correct length but fail either because the apical constriction is ovoid, funnelled or deltiform in shape, and thus not properly obturated; or because the apical foramen is placed coronal to the root-tip, so that the apparently well placed point is in fact overextended (Figure 2.1).

(2) Where a length of endodontic instrument has fractured at the root-tip, or where a sectional filling-point is misplaced (*see* Figure 1.7, page 11).

(3) Where there are obvious apical deltas or funnelling of the terminal part of the root canals.

(4) Where the apex of the root curves sharply (*see* Figure 1.8, page 11)

(5) Occasionally in the case of fractured roots when the apical fragment is to be removed, with or without the placement of an endodontic stabilizer (Figure 2.2).

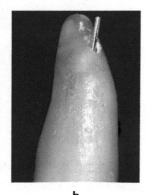
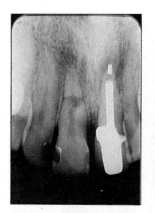
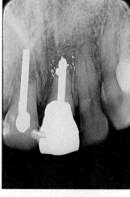

a   b

Figure 2.1 a, *Radiograph of an apparently well-filled central incisor.* **b,** *The silver point has in fact perforated the palatal aspect of the root, coronal to the apical constriction (prepared in vitro)*

a   b

Figure 2.2 a, b, *Fractured root 1| , sealed and supported by an endodontic stabilizer. The case is discussed further in Chapter 12. (Reproduced by courtesy of the Editor,* A Companion to Dental Studies*)*

(6) Where failure to drain, or repeated infection, makes impossible the completion of normal endodontic treatment (*see* Figure 7.2, page 42).

Uncontrollable chronic infection may sometimes arise from a large apical lesion. In such cases apicectomy may be the treatment of choice. However, the presence of a large apical lesion does not necessarily constitute an indication for apicectomy, and resolution may usually be expected following conventional root filling (*see* Figure 1.2, page 9). Surgical intervention may be indicated should the lesion be of such a size or appearance that biopsy is deemed desirable, or should resolution not rapidly occur following root canal therapy.

The inability to obtain drainage by way of the root canal when there is acute apical infection can afford a more urgent reason to apicect, and this should be done as soon as the acute condition has resolved as a result of drainage through the soft tissues, and/or antibiotic therapy.

When the Root Canal cannot be Instrumented or Filled to its Full Length following Removal of the Root Apex (Retrograde)

(1) Where the root canal is filled with a long metal post the removal of which is either impossible, or likely to result in fracture of the root (*see* Figure 1.10, page 12).

(2) Rarely when fractured endodontic instruments cannot be removed by means of modern endodontic techniques (Figure 2.3).

(3) Where failed root fillings cannot be removed.

(4) Where the root canal is obliterated by secondary dentine.

(5) Where there are one or more severe curvatures in the root (Figure 2.4).

When a Full-length Conventional Root Filling can be Placed, but where an Apical Seal cannot be Achieved by this Means alone (Orthograde + Retrograde)

(1) Where a tooth has died before root formation has been completed. Unfortunately, placement of a retrograde amalgam seal poses problems because the thin collar of dentine at the end of the root is extremely friable and, even if a seal can be achieved, large areas of amalgam are placed in contact with the tissues (Figure 2.5a and b). Apicectomy is a poor option in such cases and attempts should be made either to stimulate the completion of root formation or to close the apex by filling the canal with calcium hydroxide, this being followed by conventional root canal treatment. A surgical solution should be attempted as a last resort only if conservative methods fail.

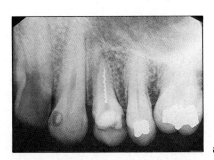

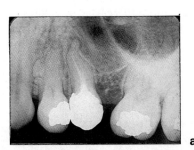

a

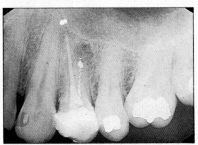

b

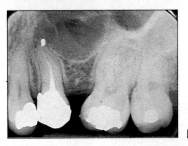

b

Figure 2.3 a, *The buccal root of ⌊4 is blocked with a fractured lentulo.* **b,** *A retrograde seal has been placed and the palatal root filled conventionally (immediately postoperative)*

Figures 2.4 a, b, *The root of ⌊5 could not be fully filled by the orthograde approach because of a double curvature and a ledge in the lower part of the canal. A seal has been effected with a retrograde amalgam. Note the proximity of the antrum (immediately postoperative)*

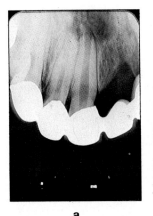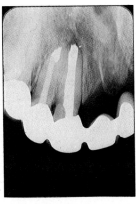

a	b

Figures 2.5 a, b, *Apicectomy of non-vital 2̲1̲\\ in an adult cleft palate patient. The bulk of the canal in ̲1̲\\ is filled with a large hand-rolled gutta-percha point (review – 19 months)*

The Repair of Root Perforations

Perforations may result either from incorrect instrumentation or from internal or external resorptions. They are usually difficult to treat, requiring a variety of approaches and the exercise of considerable ingenuity.

The subject is dealt with in Chapter 11.

Medical Reasons

Patients at risk of subacute bacterial endocarditis may have teeth root filled by conventional techniques. This will be done under antibiotic cover, usually as a one-stage procedure. However, on occasion, it may be that the operator is uncertain as to the accuracy or efficacy of the seal that he or she has achieved or is likely to achieve. In such cases an apicectomy may allow a good seal to be placed and visually checked.

Expediency·

Occasionally one or a number of teeth require to be root filled in one visit or within a short period of time. In such cases expediency may outweigh the marginally worse prognosis that is entailed by apicectomy (Figure 2.6). The same consideration may apply to patients, such as the mentally handicapped, whose treatment may have to be done under general anaesthesia, and where it is impractical to take radiographs and difficult to arrange repeated appointments.

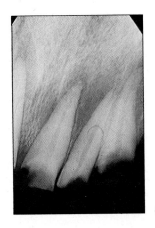

a

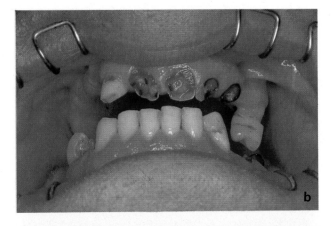

b

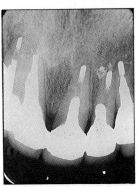

c

d

Figures 2.6 a–d, *Rehabilitation of mouth of clarinet player. 2̲1̲|̲1̲2̲3̲ were apicected in two visits. The sectional silver points were cemented with AH26. The root canals were prepared for cast gold posts at the same time. (Radiographs November 1971/September 1979). Bridge and denture are still functional (1983)*

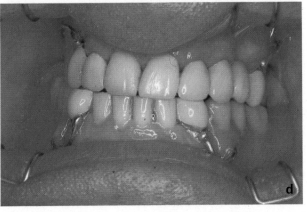

Fractured Tooth Crowns

The simplicity of use and the effectiveness of dentine pins, composite resins and glass ionomer cements allow the crowns of teeth with all but the deepest subgingival fractures to be provisionally restored so that rubber dam may be applied prior to treatment by conventional endodontic means. Apicectomy is now seldom indicated in such cases.

Crowned Teeth

The presence of artificial crowns or bridgework is seldom, if ever, a good reason for not attempting, as first choice, conventional root canal treatment. If an apicectomy is necessary, an orthograde + retrograde approach should be made. The damage done to a restoration as the result of preparing an access cavity must be set against the better prognosis when the root canal has been thoroughly cleansed and completely obturated (*see* Figure 14.1, page 95).

Chapter 3

Operative Technique: Introduction

Preoperative Assessment

The patient must always be seen on an appointment prior to that of operation in order to:

(1) undertake the necessary preparatory treatment,
(2) take a medical history,
(3) make an examination and formulate a treatment plan,
(4) explain to the patient the proposed treatment and give preoperative instructions.

Although it is chronologically correct to consider examination and treatment planning at this stage, the details will probably lack both immediacy and relevance for the inexperienced operator. This subject will therefore be dealt with in Chapter 18, following the sections on surgical technique.

Operative Procedures

The technique of apicectomy is best described in a number of clearly defined stages. These are:

(1) Preparation of an access cavity in the tooth crown (where applicable)

(2) Anaesthesia

(3) Flap reflection

(4) Removal of cortical plate and alveolar bone to reveal the root surface

(5) Isolation of the root apex*

(6) Resection of the root apex*

(7) Placement of the apical seal:
   (a) orthograde
   (b) orthograde + retrograde
   (c) retrograde

(8) Debridement of the wound

(9) Flap closure

(10) Postoperative instructions

(11) Suture removal

(12) Routine review

Each of the procedures listed above must be executed properly before the next is embarked upon. Mistakes tend to compound, exerting a domino-effect upon the subsequent stages. The advice of Jane Austen in *Pride and Prejudice* is apt:

The power of doing anything with quickness is always much prized by the possessor, and often without any attention to the imperfection of the performance.

Preparation of the Access Cavity

If the orthograde, or orthograde + retrograde techniques are to be used, an access cavity should be cut in the tooth crown, or the existing dressing removed, before the operator scrubs up.

---

*Curettage of apical tissues can be done at either stage.

Chapter 4

Operative Technique: Anaesthesia

General Anaesthesia

Vigorous bleeding can occur when an apicectomy is done under general anaesthesia; consequently, vision is obscured and it is difficult to place an uncontaminated retrograde seal. Bleeding can be reduced by infiltrating a weak solution of adrenaline (1:80 000) into the area of the wound but this requires the use of specialized general anaesthetic techniques and may be inconvenient.

Local Anaesthesia

A solution of 2% lignocaine and 1:80 000 adrenaline is an effective local anaesthetic for minor oral surgical procedures. Unless its use is dictated by the medical history, Citanest with Octapressin® is best avoided because it is not very effective in reducing bleeding and because its action is relatively short lasting. Clinical experience suggests that the depth of anaesthesia is less than when lignocaine and adrenaline is used.

Anaesthesia in the upper jaw

Anaesthesia is obtained by giving a number of buccal infiltrations and a single palatal block. A posterior superior dental block may very occasionally be required when back teeth are being treated.

Buccal infiltration

The giving of a painless injection is perhaps the most effective way of gaining the patient's early confidence. The following technique works well:

(1) Apply a topical anaesthetic ointment

(2) Use short, fine gauge needles

(3) Raise a small bleb by injecting a small increment of solution underneath the mucosa, just apical to the mucogingival junction (Figure 4.1)

(4) Leave for a minute or so then advance the needle slowly in stages through the bleb, injecting the remaining anaesthetic in increments

The final position of the needle should be such that the bulk of solution is deposited over the periosteum at a level just above the apex of the tooth (Figure 4.2).

The solution must not be injected into the lax submucosa of the buccal reflection. This will cause distension of the tissues, making it difficult to cut and reflect the flap. In addition, the depth of anaesthesia will be

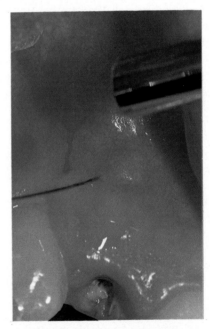

Figure 4.1 *Initial bleb of anaesthetic raised just above the mucogingival junction. Pre-extraction*

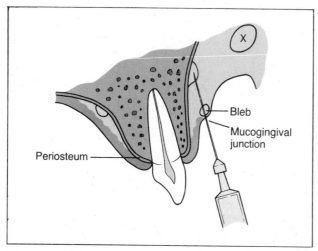

Figure 4.2 *The anaesthetic is placed over the periosteum just above the level of the tooth apex. The solution must not be injected into the lax submucosa of the buccal reflection (X)*

lessened as a result of the dispersal of solution (Figure 4.2).

The injection should be placed in three or four sites along a line just wider than the flap that is to be raised. When a single tooth is to be treated it is seldom necessary to use a total of more than 2.0 ml solution for the buccal infiltrations.

Palatal block injection

A single injection should be given, placed in relation to the tooth to be treated. Very little solution need be used, an increment of about 0.3 ml being sufficient. The injection cannot be made painless but discomfort will be lessened if the needle is placed expeditiously and the solution injected slowly with minimal pressure. The depth of palatal anaesthesia tends to reduce rapidly, often being insufficient by the time that the flap is to be sutured. It is a fine judgement, whether to repeat the injection, or to place the sutures, warning the patient that transient pain will be felt. A better option is not to place interrupted sutures, but rather to utilize a sling suture which passes around the palatal aspect of the tooth, above the sensitive palatal tissues, which are not penetrated (*see* pages 31–33).

Anaesthesia in the lower jaw

An inferior dental block should normally be given but must be supplemented by buccal and lingual infiltrations in order to obtain adequate haemostasis. If anterior teeth sited on both sides of the midline are to be apicected, an inferior dental block may be used to anaesthetize the one side, and a mental block or infiltrations the other.

Incomplete anaesthesia

Pain during the operation is distressing to both patient and surgeon. The problem usually arises only in a few specific circumstances and can generally be overcome.

Insufficient or improperly placed anaesthetic solution

Once the mucoperiosteal flap has been raised, there is no way in which the anaesthetic solution can be held against the alveolar bone, through which it must diffuse in order to be effective. It is therefore very difficult to rectify an insufficient depth of anaesthesia resulting from the initial administration of too small a quantity of anaesthetic. The same problems will arise if the flap is reflected before the proper amount of anaesthetic has fully diffused and taken effect. Pain will seldom be experienced by the patient if 5–10 minutes are allowed to elapse between the giving of the injection and raising the flap. If the injection is placed immediately after the operator has scrubbed-up, some part of the delay can be offset by the time taken in setting up the sterile handpiece, irrigation and suction.

Pain during bone removal

This will seldom occur if sufficient time elapses between the giving of the local anaesthetic and the raising of the flap. However, problems will occasionally arise when the apices of teeth (such as upper lateral incisors) are deeply placed, requiring the anaesthetic solution to diffuse through a great thickness of bone in order to be effective. Usually the buccal part of the alveolar bone can be removed without distress but drilling or curettage of the deeply placed bone that lies palatal to the root may cause pain.

In the case of a lateral incisor one or more of the following techniques can be tried.

(1) Give a high buccal infiltration. By placing the tip of the needle rather more deeply than is usual, some of the anaesthetic solution may diffuse into the infra-orbital canal, blocking the anterior superior dental nerve.

(2) Inject a small increment of anaesthetic palatally, into the incisive canal.

(3) Place an intraligamentous infiltration injection into the periodontal membrane.

(4) At one time it was normal procedure to apply a solution of cocaine on a pledget of cotton wool to the anterior floor of the nose. Although the technique is still used in ENT surgery, its use in dental practice is inadvisable on the grounds of safety and the problems of drug storage.

The use of a 4% solution of lignocaine has been described for the same purpose by Haglund and Evers (1972).

(5) If all else fails, the area of sensitivity should be identified and avoided once the root apex has been defined.

Periapical granulation tissue

Curettage of periapical granulation tissue can cause pain. This problem can often be prevented if a small quantity of anaesthetic solution is injected into the lesion immediately prior to instrumentation.

Cystic lesions

Simple dental cysts are not in themselves sensitive, but small areas of the surrounding bone cavity may be particularly so. The application of local anaesthetic solution into the bony cavity, either free or soaked on ribbon gauze, usually has little effect. Most often, all that can be done is to identify the painful area and, having decisively curetted it free of cyst lining, avoid it thereafter.

Reference

Haglund, J. and Evers, H. (1972). *Local Anaesthesia in Dentistry*. (Stockholm: Astra Läkemedical A. B.)

Chapter 5

Operative Technique: Flap Design; Reflection; Closure

Flap Design

The principles by which flaps are designed for apical surgery are few and simple.

(1) *The flap must have an adequate blood supply.* Oral mucosa is very vascular and, provided the base of the flap is not ludicrously narrow, ischaemic necrosis will not occur.

(2) *The flap must be of adequate size and fully reflected.* When a wound heals by primary closure, it unites across and not along its length, so that a long uninfected incision can be expected to heal as quickly as a short one. If a flap is inconveniently small, the operation may be poorly done as a result of insufficient access and poor visibility; in addition, the tissues are likely to be stretched or torn causing postoperative pain and slow healing.

(3) *The flap must be cleanly reflected.* Small tags of periosteum retained on the bone surface bleed, become caught in the bur during bone removal and obscure and prevent identification of small anatomical landmarks. If the flap is not cleanly reflected problems will start compounding at an early stage of the operation.

(4) *The approximated edges of the flap must lie on sound bone.* If the flap is sutured over a void, infection and breakdown of the underlying blood clot can more readily occur. As a result, healing may be delayed or, should the antrum be involved, an oroantral fistula may develop (Figure 5.1). The treatment of flap breakdown is discussed in Chapters 16 and 17.

Many flap designs have been described for use in apical surgery but most conform to one of three basic types (Figure 5.2), namely high semilunar, mid-level and envelope.

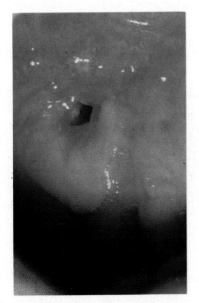

Figure 5.1 *Fistula, arising following closure of a flap across a bony void*

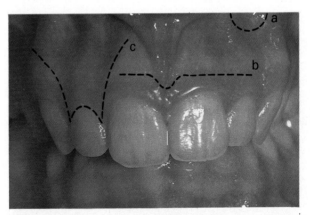

Figure 5.2 *Types of flap: a, high semilunar; b, mid-level; c, envelope*

More recently, vertical incisions finishing well short of the gingival margin have been described. These are said to allow the tissues to be reflected laterally from above the root face.

The High-level Flap

The high semilunar flap is cut in the mucosa at the level of the tooth apex. The flap is difficult to raise, affords minimal access, and cannot readily be extended. If the preoperative assessment is in error, unsuspected bone loss may cause the margins of the flap to be closed across a space. Because of the vascularity of the mucosa the cut margins may bleed freely, either during operation or postoperatively, often as a consequence of imprecise closure. The sutured margins are liable to ulcerate and healing can be slow. There are few indications for the use of the high-level semilunar flap.

A high vertical incision with lateral displacement of the mucosal tissues has been described. The incision is made immediately above the root-tip in those cases in which there is no substantial bone loss. It is claimed that access is adequate and healing rapid. I have not used this flap but would suppose that the disadvantages inherent in the high-level semilunar might equally apply.

The Mid-level Flap

Design

The horizontal incision of a mid-level flap should be made in the keratinized mucosa of the attached gingiva along a line at least 7 mm above the gingival margin. A simple straight line incision will allow enough access, provided it is of sufficient length (Figure 5.3). Closure is simplified and healing speeded if the incision is dipped to avoid cutting through the labial frenum.

The horizontal incision may be made shorter if oblique relieving incisions are cut at one or both ends (Figure 5.4); this flap is similar to the mid-level semi-lunar.

Advantages

Mid-level flaps are easy to cut and raise. They afford good access and, where relieving incisions have not been made, may readily be extended.

Closure is simple. The use of horizontal mattress sutures is sometimes advised in order to evert the margins and approximate the undersurfaces of the wound but, in most cases, simple interrupted sutures suffice (Figure 5.5a). Closure should be started centrally, subsequent sutures being placed alternately at opposite sides of the midline, working centrifugally. If suturing is started at one side of the flap, working to the other, an excess of tissue may await placement of the final suture.

Healing is usually rapid (Figure 5.5b). Early gingival recession does not occur and the subgingival margins of artificial crowns remain unexposed, in the short term. There is, however, some evidence that mucosal scarring may cause an eventual, limited recession.

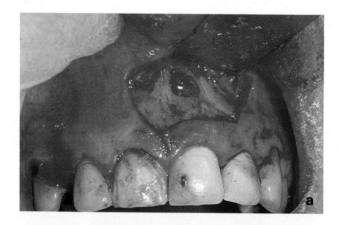

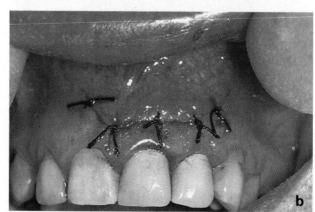

Figure 5.4 a, *Mid-level flap with relieving incisions.* **b,** *Location of the flap by means of a suture placed at each of the angles. Additional sutures prevent gaping*

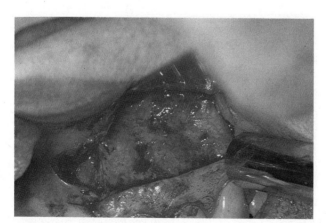

Figure 5.3 *Mid-level straight-line flap allowing good access to the root apices*

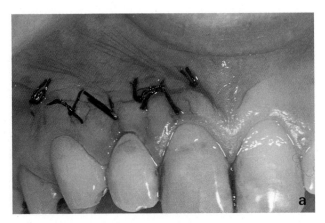

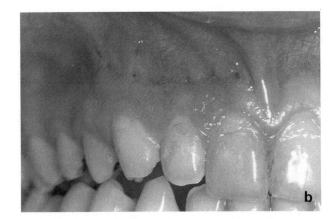

Figure 5.5 a, *Mid-level straight-line flap. Closure by means of simple interrupted sutures.* **b,** *Seven days postoperatively, following suture removal*

Disadvantages

There are several disadvantages inherent in the use of mid-level flaps.

(1) Once reflected, the flap contracts slightly and its margin tends to invert (Figure 5.6). When closing, care must be taken to untuck the edges and it may be that failure to do this causes the unsightly keloid-like scars which can develop and to which some patients may object (Figure 5.7).

(2) Occasionally, a patient will complain of neuralgic pains or numbness of the gum, a consequence presumably of cutting terminal nerve fibres. This pain can be distressing, and the patient may, for example, be unable to tolerate the pressure, upon the lip, of a sheet or blanket. The symptoms are seldom related to the extent of scarring and there is no way of determining which patients are likely to be affected.

(3) Prolonged drainage of pus from the apical lesion along the periodontal membrane can result in a loss of alveolar bone and the development of a bony dehiscence (Figure 5.16). Once apical healing has occurred and the drainage of pus has ceased as a result of apicectomy, a soft tissue union between the mucosa and root-face can be expected, but only if the pus-contaminated cementum and dentine of the root-face have been removed by root planing at the time of operation. This procedure cannot be undertaken effectively when a mid-level incision has been used, because the coronal part of the root surface remains covered by unreflected mucosa.

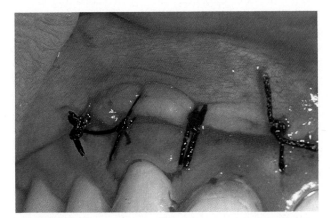

Figure 5.6 *Poorly sutured flap. The free margin on the left-hand side of the picture has inverted and this may lead to scarring*

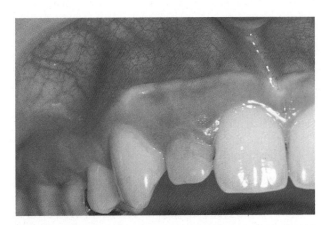

Figure 5.7 *Unsightly scarring resulting from the use of a mid-level flap*

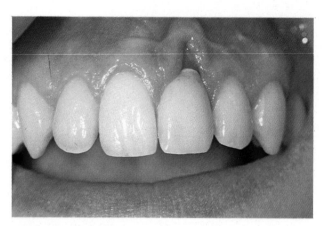

Figure 5.8 *Gingival cleft. A result of cutting and suturing a mid-level flap over a periodontal pocket. (With thanks to Mr E. Corbett for this photo of a case referred to him for treatment)*

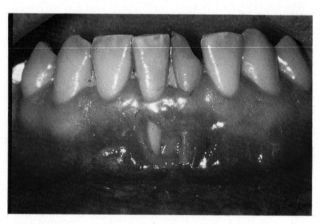

Figure 5.9 *Severe breakdown of a mid-level straight-line flap cut in the lower jaw. (With thanks to Mr B. Keiser for this photo of a case referred to him for treatment)*

(4) Attempts to suture a midline flap in a region where there is a deep periodontal pocket can result in the breakdown of tissues at the gingival crest and the formation of a cleft (Figure 5.8).

(5) If the bony lesion turns out to be unexpectedly large, or if the antrum is exposed, the line of incision may lie over a void.

(6) *In the lower jaw* the band of keratinized mucosa is seldom of sufficient width to allow mid-level incisions to be used. Even if so, the gingiva is usually thin and friable, and sutures will readily tear out because of the strong pull of the circumoral and mentalis muscles. Serious flap breakdowns, which are difficult to treat, can occur as a result (Figure 5.9). The width of the keratinized gingival band may increase towards the back of the lower jaw. Even so, the use of a mid-level flap in this part of the mouth remains inadvisable because it allows insufficient access, and because of the risk of damage to the mental nerve. *It is best routinely to raise envelope flaps when apicecting teeth in the lower jaw.*

Indications

The mid-level flap is a quick and simple procedure for use in carefully selected cases. For selection, there must be:

(1) a sufficient width of keratinized mucosa,
(2) minimal apical bone loss,
(3) no periodontal pocketing.

The principal indication for raising a mid-level flap is the need to insure against the rapid exposure of crown margins as the result of gingival recession. However, as has been stated, there is a small risk of eventual slight recession as a result of mucosal scarring.

Modification

A modification to the mid-level flap has been described. A scalloped incision is made along the junction of the keratinized gingiva and the mucosa. Unsightly scars are unlikely to develop when this flap design is used. It is claimed that healing is rapid. The flap is, however, comparatively difficult to raise.

The Envelope Flap

The envelope flap is the most time-consuming to raise and close, but offers many safeguards, particularly to surgeons who are inexperienced in apicectomy technique. The method is described in detail.

Design

The horizontal element of the flap margin is cut in the gingival crevice and usually across some part of one or more interdental papillae. Elevation is made possible by the provision of diagonal relieving incisions that extend upwards through the attached gingivae into the unkeratinized mucosa. Two relieving incisions are normally made when raising flaps in the anterior region; a single anteriorly placed relieving incision will usually allow sufficient access to posterior teeth. In carefully assessed cases where there is minimal apical bone loss and the root is straight, the horizontal incision need only be made around the neck of the involved tooth (Figure 5.10). If there is any doubt, the horizontal incision should be carried across the necks of two or more teeth (Figure 5.11a and b)

A No. 15 Swann-Morton blade is applied almost vertically into the gingival crevice so that it contacts the underlying alveolar crest. The contour of the gingival margin is followed as far as the approximal surface of the interdental papilla, which is then cut across to reach

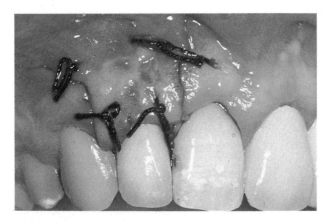

Figure 5.10 *Envelope flap involving the neck of one tooth only. The distal margin has been poorly relocated. Note that the distal relieving incision passes diagonally across the prominent canine eminence*

the approximal margin of the adjacent gingival margin. It is not necessary to extend the incision deeply into the interdental space.

The relieving incisions start at the junction between interdental papilla and the last complete gingival margin that is included in the flap (Figure 5.12).

The raising of a flap always results in the subsequent loss of a small thickness of the underlying alveolar bone. The loss is greater in the event of infection. For this reason relieving incisions should never be cut from the gingival crest (a, Figure 5.12) If such an incision is made and the wound subsequently breaks down the local destruction of the thin alveolar plate may well result in the formation of a bony dehiscence, probably associated with a gingival cleft (Figure 5.13). The breakdown of an incision-line in the interdental papilla will also cause a loss of underlying bone, but the interdental septum is sufficiently thick to accommodate such a loss and allow healing by secondary intent, without detriment.

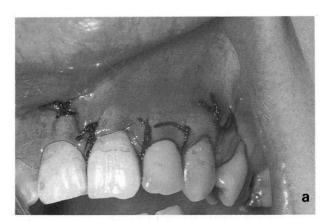

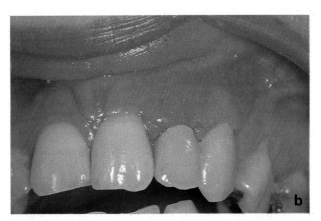

Figure 5.11 a, *Envelope flap. Apicectomy ⌊2. Note the diagonally angled suture placed across the relieving incision (see also Figure 5.10).* **b,** *Three weeks postoperatively*

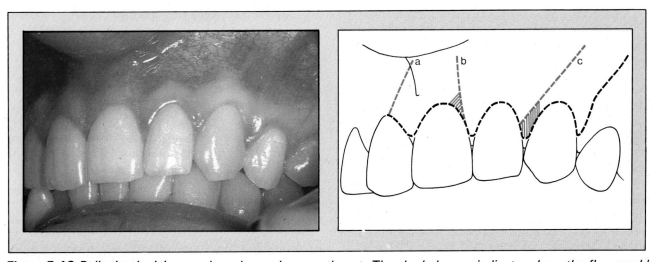

Figure 5.12 *Relieving incisions. a, b and c are incorrectly cut. The shaded areas indicate where the flap would be difficult to localize and suture*

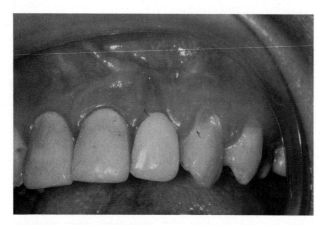

Figure 5.13 *Gingival cleft resulting from a vertical relieving incision made from the gingival crest. (With thanks to Mr B. Keiser for this photo of a case referred to him for treatment)*

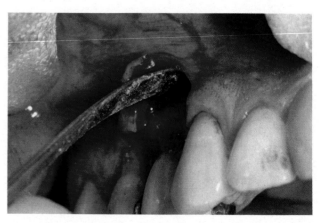

Figure 5.14 *The flap is raised with a Howarths-pattern periosteal elevator using a pushing, rather than lifting, action*

The incision should be carried upwards and sufficiently diagonally to prevent the creation of a pointed tag of gum at the margin of the flap, which can be difficult to suture in correct approximation (b, Figure 5.12). Suturing may also prove difficult if the relieving incision is too oblique (c, Figure 5.12). Once the relieving incision has been carried sufficiently high to avoid the latter hazard it should be angled more diagonally, so as to pass across rather than along the adjacent root eminences (Figures 5.10 and 5.11a). This is particularly important in the region of the prominent upper canine root, where flap breakdown can occur if the line of incision runs along the crest of the eminence. The incision is extended into the mucosa, with the knife blade being kept at all times firmly on bone.

The length of the relieving incisions is a matter of clinical judgement. In general, it is better to make them too short, since they can be extended should access prove to be insufficient. In the lower jaw, care must be taken to avoid cutting the mental nerve, and vertical relieving incisions are best not cut (or should be made short and cut with circumspection) in the area lying mesial to the first molar and distal to the canine.

Reflection

A Howarths periosteal elevator is a convenient instrument with which to reflect the mucoperiosteal flap. It should be applied with the blade almost at right angles and firmly applied to the bone. Short, isometric strokes are used to peel the periosteum from the bone using the rounded upper surface of the tip. The flap must not be levered upwards as this will cause it to tear. That part of the flap which has been cut in the mucosa tends to gape after incision and offers a convenient starting point for reflection. This should be done in a series of short progressive stages, each part of the flap being completely and cleanly raised from the bone before the next is reflected (Figure 5.14).

The flap must be reflected high enough to allow good access. However, in the anterior part of the maxilla overenthusiasm can lead to exposure of the floor of the nose which may initially be mistaken for a pathological bony lesion.

Scarring, a sinus or chronic inflammatory tissue may prevent the easy, clean reflection of the flap. In such circumstances it may be necessary to divide the restricting tissues by means of sharp dissection. In the case of scarring the scalpel blade should be directed slightly inwards so that it cuts against the bone. When granulations or scar tissue arise from a bony cavity the blade of the scalpel should again be directed slightly inward, cutting apically until the upper border of the bony deficiency is reached. Care must be taken not to perforate, or worse, resect the flap.

Once reflected, the flap may be maintained in position by the broad untoothed end of an Austin retractor. In this way the tissues are not clawed and torn and are, in addition, protected from the bur by the widest bulk of metal (*see* Figures 5.4a and 5.15).

Closure

The flap is reapproximated and sutured following surgical treatment of the root apex (to be described in subsequent chapters). A description of the suturing technique is, however, more conveniently made at this stage.

The root-face should be closely examined for bony dehiscences, before the flap is closed. Dehiscences commonly occur naturally, as a result of disproportions in root and bone morphology (Figure 5.15). There is a connective tissue attachment between the root-face and the soft tissues, and this attachment is broken when the flap is raised. The connective tissue attachment will reform following closure of the flap, provided that the torn fibres on the root-face have been neither instrumented nor otherwise damaged.

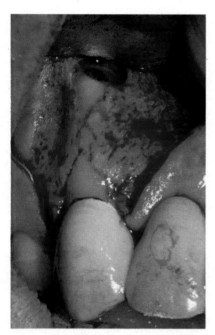

Figure 5.15 *Bony dehiscence* 3|. *There was no periodontal pocketing, and the denuded root surface is uncontaminated*

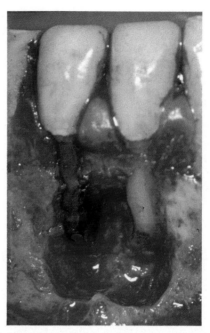

Figure 5.16 *Gross contamination of root-face and loss of buccal plate as a result of chronic apical infection*

Large bony dehiscences also commonly arise as the result of the longstanding drainage of pus from periapical lesions. The root surface is highly contaminated and is often stained and covered with calculus (Figure 5.16). All contaminated tissue must be removed from the root-face if the pocket is to be eliminated and some form of attachment regained. The root-face may be debrided by means of hand instruments or, in cases of gross contamination, with burs. Any obvious epithelial lining should be dissected from the undersurface of the flap.

Closure may be supplemented by the placement of a periodontal pack in order to conform the mucosa closely against the cleansed root surface. Provided both that an apical seal is secured and the root-face thoroughly debrided, a new attachment between the overlying soft tissues and the root-face can be hoped for. A long epithelial junction is probably formed (Figure 5.17c).

It is important to distinguish between naturally occurring dehiscences and those caused by infection, because the instrumentation of a healthy root-face may, by removing the torn periodontal fibres, jeopardize healing. The failure to recognize and debride a contaminated root-face will be equally detrimental. The subject is discussed in greater detail in Chapters 16 and 17.

Once the root-face has been considered and appropriately dealt with, the flap may be approximated and closed. A 22 mm cutting needle with 3/0 silk is suitable for most situations, although a smaller 16 mm needle is handier for thin flaps in the anterior part of the lower jaw. When the latter is being used, care must be taken

not to overtighten the suture, lest the thin silk cuts through the tissues. Resorbable catgut is rather too springy for the patient's comfort, but the newer synthetic resorbable suture materials are quite acceptable.

Closure of the flap may be considered in two stages. First, reapproximation; and second, the closure of the relieving incisions.

Reapproximation

Reapproximation must be done carefully in order to reduce the risk of recession and the unnecessary exposure of crown margins or the sensitive root surface of adjacent teeth (Figure 5.18). The use of a single sling suture or a continuous sling suture usually works well. The technique for placing such a suture is shown in Figure 5.19. The advantages of sling sutures are, first, that they exert a slight coronal displacement upon the flap thus minimizing the risk of postoperative gingival recession, and secondly, because the needle does not pass through the palatal tissues, pain is avoided at this late stage of the operation, when the effect upon the palatal tissues of the local anaesthetic may be lessening or lost.

On occasions it may not be possible to place a sling suture, and at such times an interrupted suture can be inserted across the interdental spaces. It can sometimes prove difficult to angle the needle so as to commence the lingual or palatal 'bite' at the papilla in such a way that the tip will emerge more apically through the palatal tissues. In such cases it may be more convenient to reverse the procedure, the needle being inserted

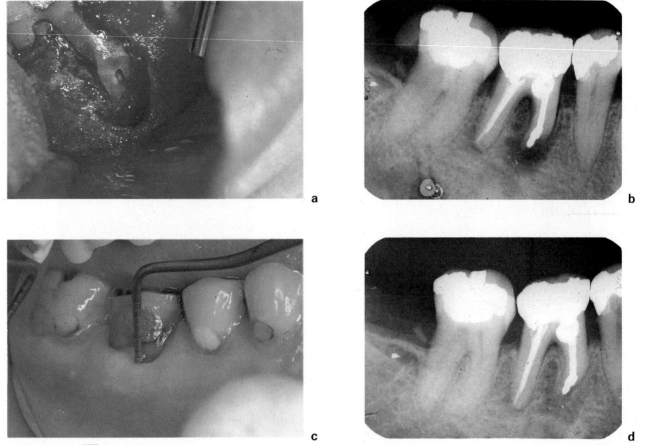

Figure 5.17 a, 6⌐ referred for apicectomy and retrograde sealing of the mesial root. Long-term chronic infection has resulted in a total loss of bony support on the buccal, mesial and distal aspects of the root. The contaminated root surface has been 'planed' with a large rosehead bur. **b,** Immediate postoperative radiograph. **c,** Review, 10 months postoperatively. Note the blanching of the gingivae and apparent absence of pocketing. **d,** Radiograph taken 10 months postoperatively

'apically', emerging from the papilla and thus producing a 'figure of eight' suture configuration (Figure 5.20). It is seldom necessary to reinforce attempts at approximation or maintenance by means of a pack. However, a pack will sometimes be used if firm adaptation of the undersurface of the flap to the root-face is required; or when periodontal manoeuvres have been undertaken as a part or in consequence of apical surgery (*see* Chapters 16 and 17).

Closure of the relieving incisions

It is usually necessary to place one or more sutures in each of the relieving incisions in order to prevent gaping. The sutures should be angled diagonally outward and downward (*see* Figures 5.10 and 5.11). In this way a slight apical displacement will occur when they are tightened. This will help to reduce the incidence of postoperative gingival recession.

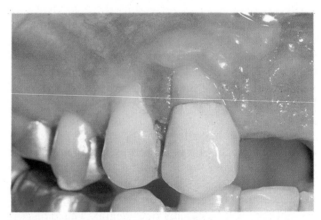

Figure 5.18 Gingival recession. The result of negligent flap approximation (referred case)

Suture removal

Sutures may be removed after 5–7 days.

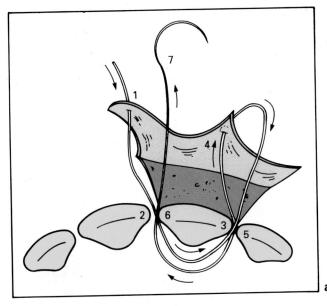

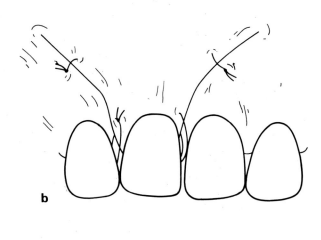

Figure 5.19 a, *The sling suture. The suture is taken: (1) through the flap from outside to inside; (2) below the contact-point, buccal to palatal; (3) behind the cingulum and then below the other contact-point, palatal to buccal; (4) through the flap from the periosteal to the outer surface; (5) beneath the contact point, buccal to palatal; (6) back around the cingulum and beneath the contact point, palatal to buccal; (7) secure with knot.* **b,** *The completed sling suture seen from the buccal*

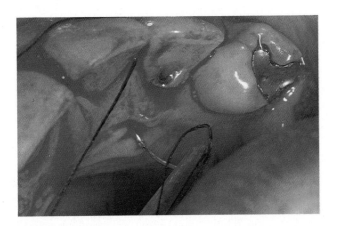

Figure 5.20 *'Figure-of-eight' suture. The needle enters the soft tissues of the palate and emerges from the interdental papilla*

Chapter 6

Operative Technique: The Root-tip; Identification and Resection

Once the tissues have been anaesthetized and a flap raised, the root-tip must be identified before it is resected and an apical seal placed.

Identification of the Root-tip

The location of the root-tip will sometimes be obvious as soon as the flap has been raised; more often its position is not immediately apparent and identification can be difficult.

The readily identified root-tip

The root-tip is readily identified in the following situations:

(1) Where the outline of the root is obvious, either beneath a thin layer of bone or exposed as a result of a dehiscence or fenestration.

(2) Where a sinus perforates the cortical plate and leads directly to the apical tissues.

(3) Where a thin layer of cortical plate overlies a granuloma or cyst. A dental probe can usually be pushed through the thin bone to identify the location and size of the underlying deficiency. Frequently the cyst lining can be exposed by peeling away the thin cortical plate with a sharp dental excavator.

(4) Where there has been a complete loss of apical bone and overlying cortical plate as a result of a long-standing granulomatous or cystic lesion, the removal of which by curettage will expose the root-tip (Figure 6.1).

In the situations listed above, a large round bur, excavator or chisel may be used to remove any remaining overlying bone so that the root-tip is exposed and

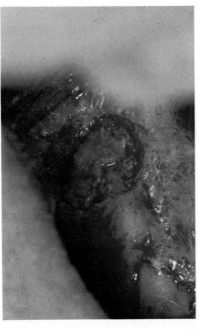

Figure 6.1 *Cystic tissue exposed immediately following flap reflection, as a result of the absence of buccal plate*

sufficient access made to allow the enucleation of apical soft-tissue lesions.

The hidden apex

A two-stage technique is best used to identify root-tips that are obscured by overlying bone. First, a small part of the root surface is exposed at a position just below the apex. Second, once this initial identification has been made, the root-tip is sculpted out in relief by careful removal of some of the adjacent alveolar bone.

Identification of the root surface

A small area of the root surface is exposed, just coronal to the apex by drilling away the overlying alveolar bone with a large round bur (No. 7–9), held in a straight handpiece. The bur is run at a high 'conventional' speed (*ca.* 10 000 rpm), and should be applied with minimal pressure so that the bone is 'painted' away in wide, shallow strokes, until the root-face is just visible (Figure 6.2a).

The root surface can be distinguished from the surrounding alveolar bone in four ways (Figure 6.2b).

(1) It is usually a different colour.
(2) It does not bleed.
(3) It is smooth, rather than granular in texture.
(4) It is surrounded by the periodontal membrane, which may be identified if the dissection has been done carefully.

When cutting, the bur and bone must be cooled and irrigated by a flow of sterile physiological saline, which is most simply applied from a large disposable plastic syringe with a blunt needle, controlled by the operating assistant.

Small round burs should not be used at this stage of bone removal because they cut deeply and tend to form pits and gouges. It is thus easy inadvertently to cut into or through the root itself, making subsequent identification of the apex difficult or impossible.

Isolation of the root apex

Once the root surface has been identified, overlying alveolar bone is removed apically, again using the large round bur (Figure 6.3). The apical length of root thus exposed should next be sculpted out in relief, by the removal of alveolar bone on its buccal aspect, and the outer parts of its mesial and distal aspects. It is usually necessary to use a smaller round bur at this stage in order to prevent damage to the roots of adjacent teeth when cutting interstitially (Figure 6.4).

Location of the apex

The length of root-tip that is isolated should be only slightly greater than the length to be resected, usually no more than 2–3 mm. *The initial exposure and identification should therefore be made as close to the apex as possible.*

Location of the apex is a skill that will develop with experience, but which can nevertheless prove difficult at any time (*see* Figures 6.3 and 6.4). The preoperative radiograph will show the approximate length and lateral inclination of the root, and this should be correlated with the angulation of the crown as seen in the mouth. Visual observation alone is an unreliable guide. For example, a misaligned tooth that has been corrected prosthetically by means of an artificial crown on an angled post and core, affords a potent trap for the

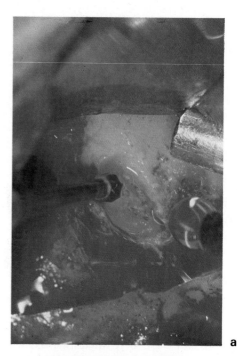

a

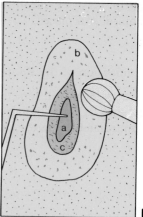

b

Figure 6.2 a, *A small area of root surface should be identified as near to the apex as possible. Bone removal is done with a large round bur.* **b,** *Diagrammatic representation. The small central area of root face (a), is a darker colour than the bone (b), and is partly covered by periodontal membrane (c). The root does not bleed and its surface feels smooth when scratched with a probe*

unwary. In such a case, the estimated location of the apex may be widely different from the true position.

Radiographs cannot indicate the depth beneath the surface at which the apex lies, so if it is possible to pass a reamer up the root canal the angle of its insertion is a useful guide.

If a tooth is very proclined, or its root abnormally curved, location of the apex can be difficult. In such cases it is best to make the initial exposure of the root surface at a relatively coronal level, where identification can be assured. The abnormally curved length may then be followed to the apex by the controlled chasing of the alveolar bone immediately overlying its surface (Figure 6.5a and c). Less damage is done in this way than by haphazardly removing quantities of apical bone.

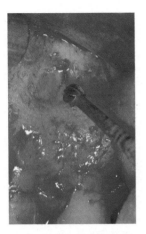

Figure 6.3 *Bone is removed to expose the upper surface of the root from the initial exposure to the apex. A large round bur is best used*

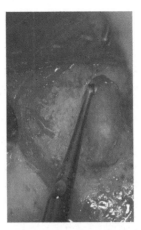

Figure 6.4 *The root-tip (seen at greater magnification) has been sculpted out in relief by using a small round bur to carefully remove sufficient surface and interstitial bone. It can be seen from both Figures 6.3 and 6.4 that the initial exposure was made too far coronally with the result that too much root has been denuded of bone*

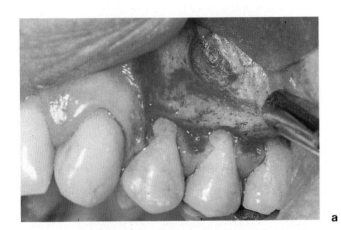

a

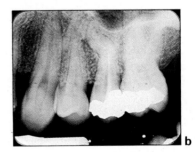

b

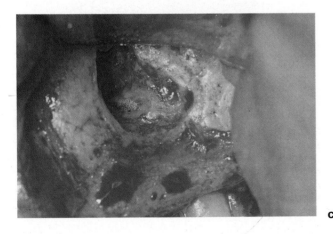

c

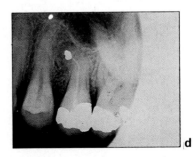

d

Figure 6.5 a, *The curved root of ⌊5 could not be filled by conventional methods. The root was initially exposed at the lowermost bend in a position where its location was certain, and the apical tip has now been identified.* **b,** *Preoperative radiograph of ⌊5.* **c,** *The resected root-tip of ⌊5. The cut face is angled forwards, a result of the root curvature. The downward and outward inclination has been superimposed by the surgeon in order to improve vision and access. Note that the retrograde amalgam seal has not yet been burnished.* **d,** *Radiograph of ⌊5, taken 7 months postoperatively*

An alternative technique?

It is tempting to try both to remove alveolar bone and resect the root apex in one manoeuvre, using a straight fissure bur. However, the technique is difficult to do well, and can cause problems. Sharp angles are cut by the bur (Figure 6.6), and blood can pool in these, so that vision is obscured. In addition, it can prove impossible to distinguish between the surfaces of bone and root cut flush with each other and, as a result, cancellous spaces in the bone may be mistaken for the root canal so that the retrograde seal is incorrectly placed (Figure 6.7a). Because the root-tip has not been isolated it may be incompletely resected (Figure 6.7b) or adjacent roots may be damaged (Figure 6.7c).

Resection of the Root-tip

The isolated root-tip is resected with a narrow fissure bur held in a straight handpiece, or in a contra-angle handpiece if access is poor.

Usually, no more than 2–3 mm of the root-tip need be cut off, namely the shortest length necessary to ensure the removal of apical deltas and to allow the root canal or canals to be seen, placed centrally in the cut face of the root, surrounded by an adequate rim of sound dentine. Sometimes, no resection need be done.

Care must be taken to ensure that the resection is carried completely through the root from buccal to lingual or palatal. If this is not done some part of the apical tip will remain in the tissues. As a safeguard the operator should always confirm that the periodontal membrane can be seen running in an unbroken ring around the cut end of the root (Figure 6.8).

Angle of resection

Occasionally, a simple horizontal resection will allow adequate access to the apical root canal – for example, when there is a large associated periapical lesion (*see* Figure 7.2, page 42). More often, visibility and access are insufficient unless the apex is resected obliquely, so that the cut root-face is angled downwards and outwards; or, in the case of back teeth, downwards, outwards and slightly forwards. There are a number of disadvantages inherent in cutting the root-tip obliquely and the angle of resection should be kept as small as possible.

Resection of the root-tip at an angle is detrimental for the following reasons:

(1) It results in the exposure of an increased number of newly cut and possibly contaminated dentinal tubules.

(2) The effective cross-sectional area of the terminal root canal is increased in geometric proportion to the obliquity of the resection. Thus, elongated canals become even more ribbon-shaped and commensurately difficult to run-out and fill with a

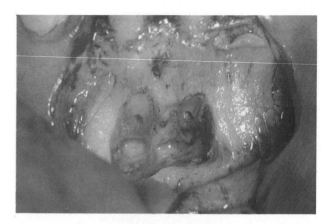

Figure 6.6 *Apicectomy 1̄|1̄. The operator has removed bone and resected both roots as a single procedure, using a flat fissure bur. The surfaces of the root-tips have been cut flush with the bone. The bony cavity is angular in contour and has been overcut, particularly lingually*

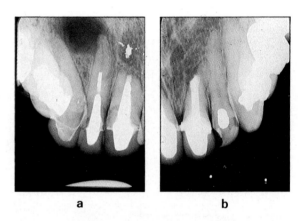

a   b

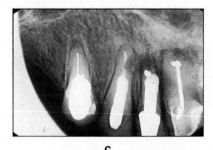

c

Figure 6.7 a, *1| has been apicected and an amalgam seal placed in the cancellous bone. 2| remains untreated.* **b,** *A perforation in the sharply curved root of |1 has been repaired with amalgam. The root-tip remains in situ.* **c,** *An 'apicectomy' of 2| and unintentionally of the mesial one half of the adjacent canine root*

retrograde sealant. Circular canals appear oval, and it is difficult to judge whether a circular filling point will seat and seal properly (Figure 6.9a).

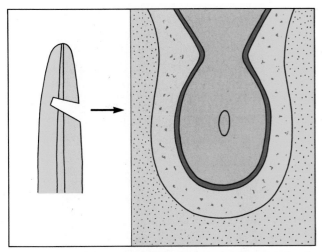

Figure 6.8 *If the root apex has been incompletely resected the periodontal ligament will be seen not to form a circle*

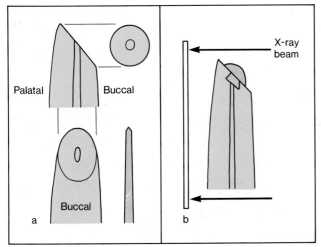

Figure 6.9 a, *A circular root canal in an obliquely-angled root-face will appear oval when viewed from in front.* **b,** *An obliquely-angled root-tip may prevent small apical areas from being seen on diagnostic radiographs*

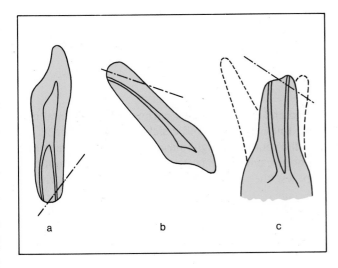

(3) Abnormal stresses may be placed on the alveolar bone by the sharply angled root end, and this may possibly delay or prevent healing.

(4) Chronic apical lesions may not be diagnosed on the follow-up radiographs because they are obscured by the superimposed, obliquely-angled root-tip (Figure 6.9b).

(5) Palatally or lingually placed foramina may not be included in the resected portion of root. This error occurs most commonly in three situations (Figure 6.10):
- (a) where an abnormally acute approach has been made in order to compensate for poor access (i.e., lower incisors),
- (b) where a tooth is retroclined (i.e., upper lateral incisors),
- (c) where a root is particularly broad buccolingually or buccopalatally (i.e., upper first molars, mesio-buccal root).

Height of resection

At one time it was advised that the apical third of the root should routinely be removed, in order to eliminate lateral canals, the majority of which were held to be located along its length. However, only when a simple retrograde seal alone is used is there a likelihood of failure as a result of toxins passing through lateral canals (*see* principles of apicectomy, Chapter 1). Even in this situation the slight risk of failure is outweighed by the harm inevitably done if one third of the root length is resected as a matter of routine (Figures 6.11 and 6.12).

A belief remains that the root should be cut down to the lowest level of the bony cavity caused by an associated pathological lesion, in order to allow complete removal of granulomatous or cystic tissue. Again, this approach is unnecessarily destructive.

Removal of Periapical Soft Tissue Pathology

It is difficult to believe that every epithelial remnant or cell can be eliminated from a bony cavity as a result of curettage or enucleation. Nevertheless, in the case of a simple dental cyst, resolution can be expected, provided that:

(1) the integrity of the epithelial sac has been destroyed,
(2) most of the epithelial cells have been removed,
(3) the toxic stimulus from the root canal has been eliminated by the placement of an apical seal.

Figure 6.10 *The apical foramina may not be included in the resected section of root-tip in the following situations:* **a,** *where the resection is too oblique,* **b,** *where the tooth is severely retroclined,* **c,** *where the roots are particularly broad buccopalatally or bucco-lingually*

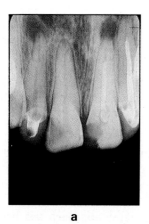
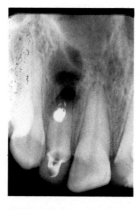

a

Figure 6.11 *About one half of the root length of the 2] has been resected, needlessly destroying support. The root canal remains unfilled and the apical seal is excessively large*

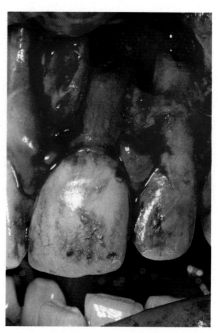

Figure 6.12 *Unacceptable reduction in root length, the result of several apicectomies*

The likelihood of a favourable outcome should not, however, be made an excuse for a sloppy surgical technique and every attempt must be made to remove all the pathological periapical soft tissue at the time of operation. This affords additional advantages.

(1) The root-tip is clearly exposed.
(2) Haemorrhage is reduced and can be further diminished by packing the bony cavity with ribbon gauze soaked in a solution of 2% lignocaine and 1:80 000 adrenaline (*see* Figure 7.5, page 44).
(3) Debris, such as amalgam, is less likely to be retained in a clean cavity that can readily be inspected and washed out.

It is often necessary to curette away some of the apical granulations immediately after the buccal plate has been removed in order to see and expose the root-tip (*see* Figure 7.2a and b, page 42). However, the bulk of the lesion is usually more easily curetted or enucleated once the root-tip has been resected. If access is insufficient it is better to judiciously remove more alveolar bone, rather than resect the root to a lower level.

If possible, the lesion should be removed intact rather than piecemeal. Large, round excavators or the spoon-shaped end of a Mitchell's trimmer are useful for the purpose. Initially the tissues may be peeled away from the cavity wall by pushing with the convex, non-cutting side of the excavator blade (a, Figure 6.13). However, once they have been released as far as the back wall of the bony cavity, this action is ineffective and the blade must be inverted and used with a scooping movement (b, Figure 6.13). Granulations or cyst-lining at the back and sides of the root are difficult and tedious to remove, especially where the space between tooth and alveolar bone narrows coronally (c, Figure 6.13). Here it is a matter of determination and ingenuity, and a variety of instruments can be brought into use, including the

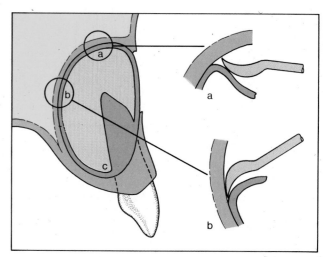

Figure 6.13 *Removal of apical soft-tissue lesions. A prising action may be used at (a), but a scooping action with the opposite face of the excavator or curette blade is required at (b). It is difficult to remove tissue from the region marked (c)*

bladed end of the Mitchell's trimmer, periodontal curettes, fine excavators and a sickle or Briault probe.

If the root of a neighbouring vital tooth extends into the bony cavity, it is best to avoid curetting around its apex lest the vascular bundle be damaged and vitality lost.

A substantial sample of the lesion wall and contents should be preserved in a 10% solution of formol saline, for histological examination and report.

Chapter 7

Operative Technique: The Apical Seal

In Chapter 2, three principal types of apical seal were described. These were:

Orthograde

Orthograde + Retrograde

Retrograde

The techniques are summarized in Figure 7.1.

The Orthograde Apical Seal

After the root-tip has been resected, the apical part of the canal must be sealed in order to prevent the egress of toxins into the tissues. If the root canal is patent it should, whenever possible, be filled with a cemented gutta-percha point or points.

The simple method of placing a gutta-percha point or

points, described below, also forms the basis for the combined orthograde + retrograde technique.

An access cavity will have been cut prior to operation. Preparation of the canal is a quick and simple procedure. There is no need or reason to instrument to an exact length and the passage of the reamers through the apicected root-tip can be readily observed and controlled (Figure 7.2c).

The apical part of the canal should be *reamed* to a circular shape, the more coronal parts *filed* to remove debris. If K-type files are used, both procedures can be undertaken with the same instrument. The files (retained for safety in a chained clip) should be used sequentially, the canal being repeatedly irrigated, conveniently with local anaesthetic solution applied through a fine bore needle.

Reaming and filing may be ceased when the canal is

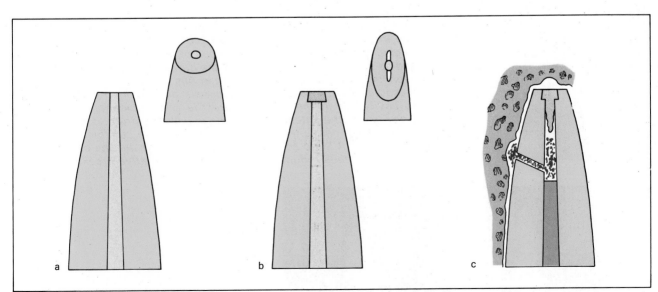

Figure 7.1 *Diagrammatic representation of the three types of apicectomy technique.* **a,** *Orthograde,* **b,** *orthograde + retrograde,* **c,** *retrograde*

41

free of debris, and when the apical foramen is seen to be circular in shape and bordered by sound dentine. However, if the root-tip has been cut obliquely, an accurate assessment of circularity can be made only when the point is fitted.

When instrumentation has been completed, a suitably sized filling point is tried in, being pushed until it passes through the apical foramen to wedge firmly. If the fit of the point is poor the canal should be reamed to a larger size in an attempt to make the apical foramen more circular. If this cannot be done a combined ortho-grade + retrograde technique will have to be used.

The chosen filling point is next removed from the canal which is irrigated, then dried with paper points. A quick-setting cement such as Tubliseal (Kerr) is applied on a reamer rotated in reverse direction until the canal is well filled; and the coated point is firmly seated. When the cement has set the point is cut flush with the root surface by means of a *new* scalpel blade (Figure 7.2d).

The smooth surface that can be achieved in this way is illustrated in Figure 1.4, page 10. The cut point may be warm burnished to give an optimal marginal seal (Figure 7.4).

A heated instrument must not be used to sear the point, because this will cause it to drag, elongate and narrow so that the apical seal is jeopardized. Finally, the adaptation of the cut point to the canal should again be checked. If there is any doubt that the fit is good, a retrograde seal must be placed. Closure of the flap (Figure 7.2e) has been described previously.

There are several possible variations in the 'ortho-grade' filling technique described above. The canal can, for example, be obturated with laterally condensed gutta-percha, gutta-percha points or thermoplasticized gutta-percha. However, in each case the basic apicec-tomy procedure is the same.

The likelihood that the cement seal will dissolve in the tissues over a period of time might be thought a good

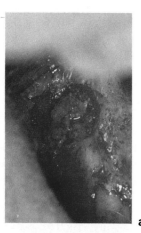
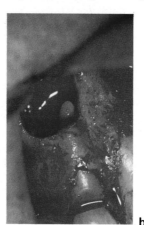
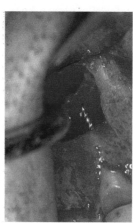
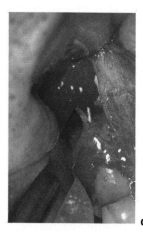

a   b   c   d

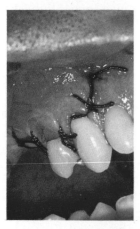

e

Figure 7.2 *Surgical endodontic treatment of a non-vital 4 ⌋. The patient had been referred because of facial swelling. The release of pus could not be obtained by way of the root canals, and initial treatment included a drainage incision in the buccal mucosa plus antibiotic therapy.* **a,** *Apical pathological soft tissue revealed as a result of flap reflection.* **b,** *Buccal root exposed as a result of the removal of the soft tissue. The palatal root has also been identified but cannot be seen in this view.* **c,** *Both root-tips have been resected horizontally, and the canals directly instrumented via an access cavity cut in the crown. Note the communication between the cystic cavity and the anterior part of the maxillary antrum.* **d,** *Gutta-percha points have been cemented into both roots and are cut flush with a new scalpel blade.* **e,** *A large envelope flap ensures that the line of closure lies on sound bone, thus reducing the risk of postoperative breakdown*

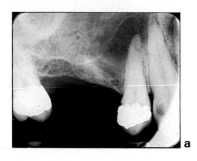
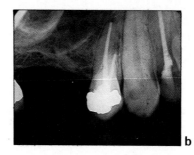

a   b

Figure 7.3 *Radiographs of case illustrated in Figure 7.2.* **a,** *Preoperative,* **b,** *11 months postoperative*

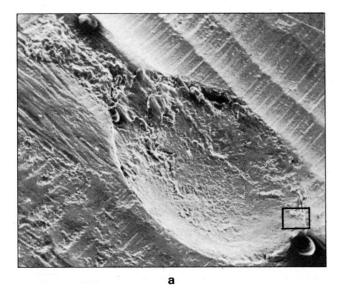
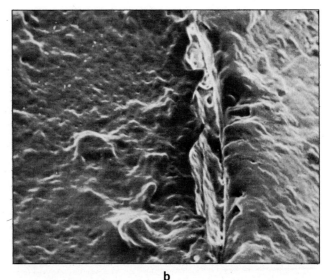

a   b

Figure 7.4 *Size 70 gutta-percha point cemented prior to resection of the root-tip with a fissure bur, and warm-burnished after resection. SEM photomicrograph of replica. The surface of the seal is smooth, but burnishing has failed to eliminate the interfacial deficiency between the point and the root canal wall.* **a,** *Field of view 2 mm,* **b,** *field of view 150 μm. (Photomicrographs taken by courtesy of Professor Alan Boyde, University College, London)*

reason for not using the orthograde apicectomy technique. In practice, cement loss does not seem to be a problem and the simplicity of the method is convenient, particularly when access is poor and the placement of a retrograde seal might prove difficult.

Root filling prior to apicectomy

It is a common practice to root fill teeth on a visit prior to apicectomy. There are several reasons why this technique cannot be recommended.

(1) Unless the filling is placed immediately prior to operation there is a likelihood that acute apical infection will supervene. Antibiotics are sometimes overprescribed to prevent this.

(2) Unless the root filling is precisely done, the point is likely to be a poor fit within the canal and, consequently, a large area of cement will be exposed to the tissues following apicectomy.

If the root filling is properly done in order to ensure a wedge-fit of the point, far more time will be spent than if instrumentation of the canal were to be undertaken at the time of operation.

(3) When the root-tip is resected, the cut end of the gutta-percha filling point is roughened and the cement disrupted by the action of the bur. In addition, gutta-percha may be smeared across the root-face making it impossible to check the adequacy of the apical seal.

If the technique is used, then following resection the gutta-percha seal should be adapted against the canal wall by means of warm-burnishing (Figure 7.4).

The Orthograde Filling + Retrograde Seal

It is necessary to reinforce an orthograde filling with a retrograde seal in the following circumstances.

(1) When, following instrumentation and trial placement of the filling point, it is seen that the terminal part of the canal has not been reamed to a circular cross-section.

(2) When the apical length of root canal is observed immediately following the resection to be so irregular in cross-section that there is no purpose in attempting to ream it to a circular shape.

(3) When a failed root filling is to be retained and corrected surgically rather than being removed and replaced.

Before discussing techniques of retrograde filling it is necessary to consider briefly the nature of the retrograde apical seal. There is no doubt that amalgam is not entirely well tolerated by the tissues, and this is discussed further in Chapter 14. Currently much research is being undertaken on the development of a more compatible material. Nevertheless, at present the literature suggests that the best results are still obtained from the use of spherical, zinc-free amalgam. Zinc-free amalgam is advised, not because of the fear of moisture contamination (the cavity into which the seal is packed should be blood-free), but because it is considered that zinc may be toxic to the tissues. It is generally recommended that the depth of the seal should be at least 3 mm, and even then microleakage may occur. Every attempt must be taken, therefore, to ensure that all of the root canal beneath the amalagm seal is

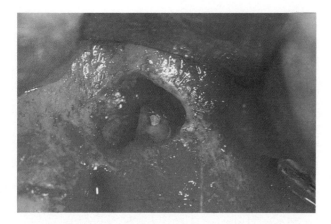

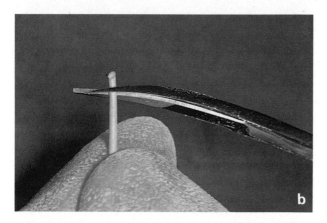

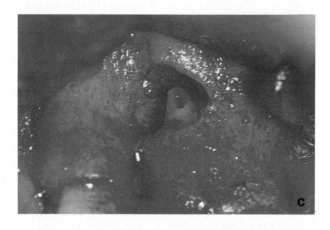

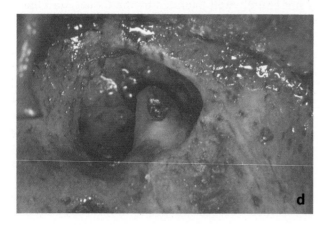

cleansed of noxious debris and obturated with a suitable material. This will be discussed later.

For a more detailed consideration of the nature of the apical retrograde seal, readers are referred to the chapter on 'Surgical Endodontics' in *Endodontics in Clinical Practice* by Harty.

1. The imperfectly reamed apical canal

In the simple orthograde apicectomy technique the apical part of the root canal is reamed to a circular cross-section, prior to cementing a conventional filling point. Occasionally, the trial point will be found to fit imperfectly, because irregularities in the shape of the apical root canal have not been completely eliminated. If further reaming is either not possible or is unlikely to effect an improvement, the apical seal must be secured with a retrograde filling.

The technique is simple (Figures 7.5 and 7.6). The uncemented, ill-fitting point is cut flush with the root surface and is then withdrawn from the canal. A further 3 mm is cut from its tip, maintaining the obliquity of section, and the shortened point is cemented into the canal with a quick-setting sealant such as Tubliseal. When the cement has set, an apical cavity is prepared by drilling out the upper 3 mm of the root canal with a small, round bur, at the same time freshening the dentine walls. It is easier and quicker to drill cement from the canal in this way than it is to cut away the end of a full-length cemented gutta-percha or silver point.

The apical part of the canal will be slightly cone-shaped as a result of reaming and no positive attempt need be made to prepare undercuts for retention of the amalgam seal.

Alternatively, the amalgam seal can be condensed against the shortened *uncemented* point which is then withdrawn from the canal and cemented back into position. The procedure is quick because there is no need to wait for cement to set before preparing and filling the apical cavity. However, because of the viscosity of the sealant, the gutta-percha point can rarely be fully seated (Figure 7.8) and there is also a risk that the apical amalgam filling may be dislodged.

The orthograde + retrograde techniques that have just been described are not elective, but rather are salvage operations undertaken to correct what would otherwise

Figure 7.5 *Orthograde + retrograde apicectomy* ⌊2. **a,** *The gutta-percha point has been cut flush with the root-face, but does not properly fit the reamed canal.* **b,** *A length is cut from the tip of the point.* **c,** *An apical cavity has been prepared following recementation of the shortened point.* **d,** *Completed, burnished silver-amalgam seal. The bony cavity was packed with ribbon gauze moistened with local anaesthetic solution, prior to placement of the amalgam. Note the relatively blood-free field*

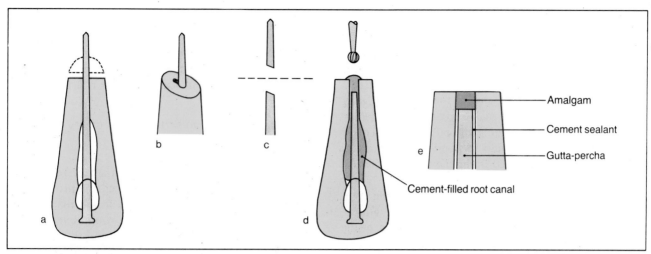

Figure 7.6 *Diagrammatic representation of the orthograde + retrograde technique. In* **(d)** *the coronal length part of the root canal is shown largely filled with cement. This space may be obturated with accessory gutta-percha points, using a lateral condensation technique*

be an unsuccessful apicectomy. They are necessary because the surgeon has failed to recognize, at an early stage of the operation, that an irregularly shaped apical root canal could not be successfully reamed to a circular cross-section to which a filling point would accurately fit. As a consequence, the apical canal will have been unnecessarily enlarged by reaming, with the result that an excessive amount of amalgam is placed in contact with the tissues (compare the size of the apical amalgam seals shown in Figures 7.7 and 7.8).

The apical part of a root canal should be enlarged by reaming only if there is a good chance of rendering it *circular in cross-section so that a well-fitting orthograde point can be sealed.*

2. The irregular canal

No attempt should be made to ream the apical part of a root canal that is obviously grossly irregular in its apical cross-section. Instead, the whole canal should be *filed* clean of debris, and the largest point(s) chosen that just pass through the foramen (Figure 7.9). The filling is cut short by 3 mm, and an amalgam seal placed using one of the techniques described above. Again, lateral condensation or thermoplastic techniques are very suitable.

Dinsdale and Holmes (personal communication) have suggested the use of a proprietary, calcium hydroxide based, sub-lining material to obturate the cleansed canal. The paste is readily spun into position and sets rapidly. The apical cavity can be prepared and the amalgam seal packed against a sound base with little delay. Amalgam powder can be mixed with the unset paste to increase the radiopacity.

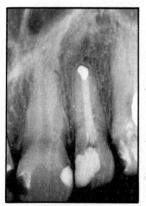
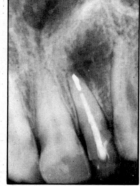

Figure 7.7   **Figure 7.8**

Figure 7.7 *Radiograph of case illustrated in Figure 7.5, 1 year postoperatively. Note the size of the amalgam seal in comparison with that shown in Figure 7.8, where the apical root canal had not been reamed prior to placement of the amalgam*

Figure 7.8 *Apicectomy ⌐2, immediately postoperatively. The apical root canal was not reamed and the seal is therefore small in surface area. The gutta-percha point was cemented after the amalgam was packed, and is not fully seated*

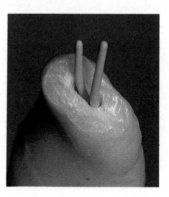

Figure 7.9 *Partial obturation of an irregular canal, prior to placement of the apical amalgam seal*

3. The failed root filling

The indications for apicecting an unsuccessful root filling were discussed in Chapter 2. Only rarely is it sufficient simply to resect the tip of the root; usually the fit of the obturating point will be found to be imperfect. In such cases the terminal 3 mm of the root filling may usually be cut away, the coronal length being retained as a base against which the amalgam seal is condensed. A grossly ill-fitting point should, if possible, be removed so that a properly condensed filling may be placed prior to securing the apical seal.

The removal of the apical part of an existing root filling can be difficult and time-consuming. Gutta-percha seldom cuts cleanly, small resilient tags being pulled from its surface by the bur. These tags may get in the way when the amalgam seal is being placed and must be cut free with a small excavator or teased out with a Briault probe.

If a silver point has to be cut down, care must be taken that the bur does not skid into the softer dentine, perforating the root. New steel burs can be used to cut metal, but they blunt rapidly and must frequently be replaced. Small tungsten carbide burs such as those supplied with the Kavo apicectomy handpiece are useful (Figure 7.10), or alternatively a round diamond or tungsten carbide bur may be used in a high-speed (double red) 'conventional' handpiece.

The Simple Retrograde Seal

The placement of a simple retrograde seal is indicated when the root canal cannot be instrumented to accommodate the fit of an orthograde filling. The method of placing the amalgam described below is also applicable to the final stage of the orthograde + retrograde technique.

Identification of the root canals

The entrances of narrow, uninstrumented canals are often obscured by smeared dentine, following resection of the root-tip. They may be located and their entrances made patent by careful searching with a Briault probe.

Preparation of the apical cavity

The bur

The apical cavity is best cut with a small, round bur. The bur tip can be used in the manner of a probe to feel for the canal entrance, into which it will readily drop when rotated. Once in the canal, a round bur will tend to follow the path of least resistance and this facilitates the running-out of narrow crevice-like canals with minimal risk of perforation. It is seldom necessary to use a size greater than No. ½ (Figure 7.11), and this may be inconveniently large for teeth with particularly narrow roots, such as lower incisors (Figure 7.12).

Inverted-cone burs should not be used. They afford none of the advantages of the round bur and are likely to create perforations (see Figure 7.13).

The handpiece

If the apical cavity is to be cut with precision, the bur is best rotated at relatively low speed. By using a standard contra-angle bur in a childrens-head handpiece, an extra length of shank is exposed, which affords a

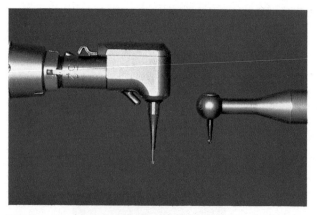

Figure 7.10 *A standard bur in a childrens-head handpiece (left) usually allows adequate access. A special apicectomy handpiece with integral tungsten carbide bur is available (right) and is sometimes useful*

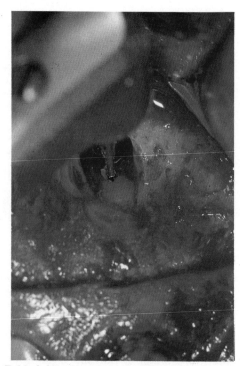

Figure 7.11 *A No. ½ round rosehead bur is optimal in size and shape for preparing most apical cavities*

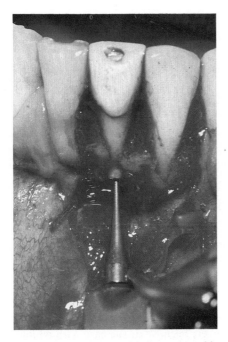

Figure 7.12 *A round bur in a childrens-head handpiece is satisfactorily being used to prepare an apical cavity in a lower incisor, despite the poor access. Note that even this small bur is almost too wide to be used in the narrow root*

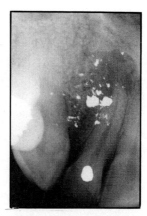

Figure 7.14 *Postoperative radiograph of an attempted apicectomy 2⌋ (referred case). The amalgam 'seal' is liberally dispersed throughout the tissues*

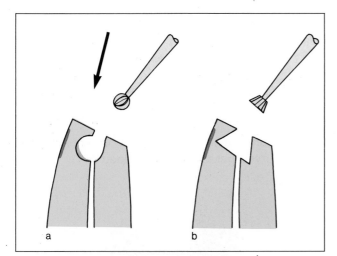

Figure 7.13 a, *The apical cavity should be cut from as near vertical as possible (see arrow). An oblique approach is sometimes used to prepare a floor (blue line) against which the amalgam is condensed. However, the risk of root perforation (indicated by the red line) is increased, particularly if an inverted cone bur is used* **(b)**

be made with the standard handpiece. Second, where the integral tungsten carbide bur is used to drill metal from the root canal. The shortness of the system is, however, sometimes a hindrance, either because the handpiece head lies so close to the root apex that vision is obscured, or because it impacts against the bony cavity wall preventing the bur from reaching deeply placed roots. In addition, the smallest round bur currently available is often inconveniently large.

The cavity

The apical cavity should be cut with the bur applied as nearly as possible down the long axis of the root canal. An oblique approach is sometimes advocated in order to prepare an angled palatal or lingual wall against which the amalgam can be condensed. However, if this is done the risk of perforation is increased (Figure 7.13).

The circumference of the canal wall should be 'freshened' with the bur to a depth of about 3 mm. Narrow fissure-shaped canals must be run out and sufficiently widened to allow the amalgam to be placed and properly condensed. When two canals lie close together in the same root it is sensible to drill out the narrow bridge of dentine that lies between them lest unseen microscopic fissures remain unfilled. Failure to do this is the probable cause of many poor results, particularly in upper premolar teeth.

It is usual to prepare undercuts for the retention of the apical filling. These need be minimal and should be made by a slight sideways movement of the bur. If the tip of the bur is used there is a risk of overcutting and perforating the root (Figure 7.13a).

Placement of the amalgam

The amalgam alloy

Patients who are referred for further treatment often exhibit a 'gunshot' or 'snowstorm' appearance on their

valuable increase in access and visibility (Figures 7.10, 7.11 and 7.12).

A special apicectomy handpiece with a miniature head is available (Kavo Ltd, Figure 7.10) and is very useful in two situations. First, where there is an insufficient depth of sulcus to allow a near vertical approach to

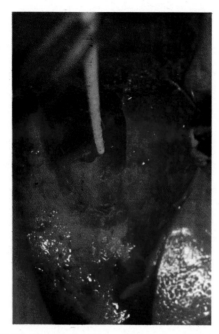

Figure 7.15 *A paper point should be used to dry the washed apical cavity before the amalgam seal is packed*

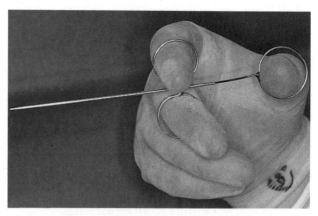

Figure 7.16 *A 'home-made' amalgam carrier. The ringed handles allow manipulation with one hand*

periapical radiographs – a result of the inaccurate dispersal of amalgam in the bone and soft tissues (Figure 7.14). This is indicative of a careless operating technique, but more importantly it may affect the well-being of the patient. The effect of amalgam on the tissues will be discussed in Chapter 14. It is sufficient at this stage to state that the amalgam seal must be contained within the root canal. Particles of amalgam should never be dispersed in the surrounding tissues. In addition, every effort must be made to ensure that the size of the apical seal (and thus the area of amalgam in contact with the tissues) is as small as possible.

Spherical alloy is a useful material in the hands of an experienced operator. It can be well condensed into deep or irregular cavities, with minimal packing pressure. However, because of the ease with which it flows it is very easy to overfill the root canal. Care must be also taken to ensure that the periodontal membrane and bone spaces do not become permeated with metal.

Debridement of the apical cavity

The apical cavity will be contaminated with blood and debris and must be washed out (with local anaesthetic solution applied through a fine-bore needle), and dried with paper points before the amalgam is placed (Figure 7.15).

Control of haemorrhage

The amalgam seal should be packed, uncontaminated, in a field free from moisture and blood.

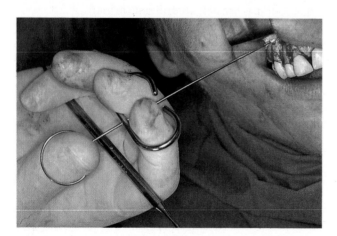

Figure 7.17 *Placement of the amalgam increment with an 'Endogun'*

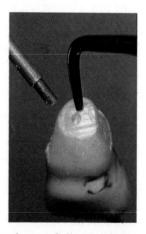

Figure 7.18 *The bore of the amalgam carrier may be wider than the apical cavity. The plugger must be narrower*

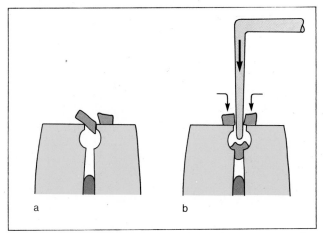

Figure 7.19 *If the increment of amalgam cannot be placed directly into the apical cavity it should lie centrally on the cut root-face* **(a)**. *Packing pressure must be applied directly into the apical cavity* **(b)**, *further portions of amalgam being fed in from the side*

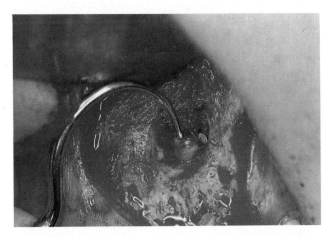

Figure 7.20 *A 'Thymosin' instrument is being used to feed and pack the amalgam increment into the apical cavity. The ball-end of the instrument is smaller than the apical cavity*

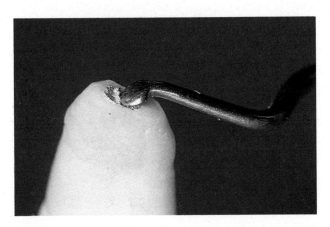

Figure 7.21 *The surface of the partly-set amalgam is carved flat with a large round excavator, inverted; prior to burnishing*

Bleeding will seldom cause problems if bony cavities are packed with ½″ wide ribbon gauze soaked with local anaesthetic solution containing 1:80 000 adrenaline (Figure 7.5). However, in the absence of a periapical lesion such packing is rarely possible and haemorrhage from newly-cut cancellous bone may often be troublesome. Bleeding can usually be controlled by efficient suction. Fine sucker tips are helpful but they quickly become blocked, particularly when used with high volume/low vacuum aspiration systems. Haemorrhage occurring from a wide area of cut bone can sometimes be reduced by the application of bone wax, though this material is difficult to place and maintain. Localized haemorrhage can often be staunched by the wedging or burnishing of bone across the bleeding point.

The amalgam carrier

Many types of carrier have been designed to facilitate placement of the amalgam into the apical cavity. Because of the difficulty in constructing a robust and reliable angled tip, most are straight and must be applied at an angle to the long axis of the root canal.

An inexpensive carrier can be made from 0.045-inch (1 mm) internal diameter orthodontic stainless steel tubing and 0.045-inch (1 mm) gauge wire (Figure 7.16). The ringed finger and thumb grips allow the carrier to be loaded and manipulated with one hand, leaving the other free to maintain reflection of the flap. The barrel is sufficiently long for sections to be cut from its tip when blockage occurs, but not so long as to unduly magnify tremor. A ready-made version is available commercially* (Figure 7.17). It can be seen that the bore of the carrier is wider than the average apical cavity (Figure 7.18). Narrower carriers can be made, but are not entirely satisfactory, being difficult to load and prone to blockage.

Placement and condensation of the amalgam

It is seldom possible to place a complete increment of amalgam directly into the apical cavity, and usually some will lie centrally on the surface of the cut root-tip (Figure 7.19a). A small plugger should be used to condense down through the central part of this surface amalgam directly into the apical cavity, the remaining portion being fed in from the sides (Figure 7.19b).

The plugger *must be narrower* than the apical cavity (Figure 7.19b). A 'Thymosin' instrument (Figure 7.20) or the pointed end of a Baldwin burnisher are useful. If required, smaller pluggers can be made by modifying old dental probes or other hand instruments. Amalgam inadvertently forced down the periodontal membrane or into cancellous bone spaces can seldom completely

*Endogun. Prima-Quality Instruments, 23 Faris Barn Drive, Woodham, Weybridge, Surrey KT15 3DZ

be removed. In order to prevent this happening, a bulk of amalgam should never be allowed to build up on the surface of the cut root-tip, and gross excess must be removed before a further increment is placed. Similarly, packing pressure should never be applied anywhere other than directly into the root canal.

When the apical cavity has been slightly overfilled, the amalgam should be allowed partly to set before it is carved flush with the root-face. This can be done with a large round excavator, used inverted with a chisel-like action so as to cut a flat surface (Figure 7.21). Finally, the amalgam surface should be gently burnished (Figure 7.22).

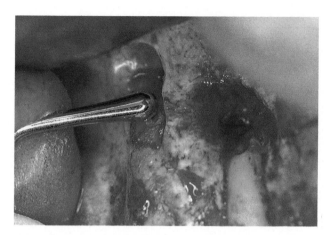

Figure 7.22 *Pear-shaped burnisher being used to burnish the partly-set amalgam seal*

The unfilled apical canal

In many instances there may be a substantial length of unfilled root canal lying apical to the obstruction that has made necessary the provision of an apical amalgam seal (*see* Figure 7.25). Every attempt must be made to obturate this empty space. It is not a good idea to try to plug amalgam into the void. It is unlikely that the amalgam will be adequately condensed, with the risk that the continued microleakage of the noxious material that remains in the uncleansed canal may cause the apicectomy to fail. Instead, once the apex of the tooth has been resected and the apical cavity prepared, the empty canal should be filed clean, using a file bent at its end, so as to get access (Figure 7.23). The canal is irrigated with local anaesthetic solution applied through a bent needle (Figure 7.24). The cleansed length of apical canal is then obturated prior to placing a 3 mm amalgam retrograde seal. A number of methods for filling the coronal lengths of canal have been described, including the use of thermoplasticized gutta-percha. Simplest is to puddle a sealant such as Tubliseal into the cleansed canal, and then to tease in a few short pieces of gutta-percha point, prior to recutting the apical cavity and placing the amalgam seal which can now be well condensed (Figure 7.25).

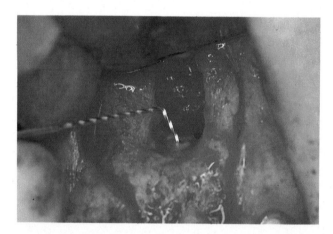

Figure 7.23 *A file, the tip of which is bent at right angles, is being used to cleanse the unfilled length of root canal*

Debridement of the Wound

Bony cavities should routinely be packed with a length of 13 mm (half-inch) wide ribbon gauze before the amalgam is placed. Loose particles of alloy will be removed when the gauze is released from the cavity, which should then be thoroughly washed out and checked visually. Amalgam fragments lying over the periodontal membrane or on cancellous bone can usually be washed off, providing that they have not been subjected to pressure. Fragments that do not wash off should be picked out with the tip of a probe, under copious irrigation. Excavators or curettes should not be used because they tend to compress the material further into the tissues.

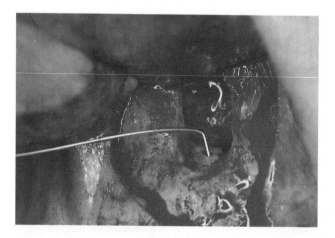

Figure 7.24 *The instrumented apical canal is further cleansed by means of irrigation with local anaesthetic applied through a fine bent needle*

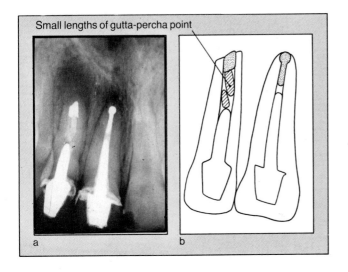

Small lengths of gutta-percha point

a   b

Figure 7.25 a, b, *Apicectomy* 21]. *Pieces of gutta-percha were placed in the patent canal* 2] *to prevent over-packing and to allow proper condensation. This was not done* 1], *which is slightly overfilled as a result*

The undersurface of the flap and the upper surface of the alveolus must be checked for debris before closure. Small retained pieces of amalgam are easily overlooked, particularly when they are wedged in the upper part of the flap reflection. Amalgam tattoos are a frequent consequence. Treatment of the condition is discussed in Chapter 17.

Closure

Closure has been described in Chapter 4. The patient must be advised not to raise the lip to view the wound lest the sutures tear through the swollen tissues.

Postoperative Radiographs

A postoperative radiograph should be taken prior to or immediately following placement of the sutures. If an operative error is apparent it is usually best to correct it straight away.

Reference

Harty, F. J. (1990). Surgical endodontics. In *Endodontics in Clinical Practice*, pp. 224–293. (London: Wright)

Chapter 8

Operative Technique: Postoperative Recovery

Prescription of a postoperative chlorhexidine mouth rinse, to be used twice a day, may help to reduce the incidence or severity of wound infection, and thus of postoperative discomfort. A chlorhexidine mouth rinse taken prior to the operation may also be of value in this respect. Despite these precautions, pain, swelling, and bruising may occur following periapical surgery, and often the severity bears no relation to the difficulty of the operative procedure. Pain can normally be controlled by mild analgesics. Aspirin works well, particularly if given to the patient immediately postoperatively, after bleeding has stopped and clotting has taken place, but before the effect of the local anaesthetic has worn off. Also, the degree of pain appears to be related principally to the amount of early trauma to which the patient has been subjected, particularly the handling of the soft tissues during the raising of the flap. The implications are obvious. Swelling usually develops during the day after surgery and should be well resolved after 5 days. Bruising lasts longer.

It is sensible to administer antibiotics (ideally preoperatively) when a large intrabony lesion is to be enucleated, in an attempt to prevent infection and breakdown of the blood clot. Simple apicectomies for a healthy patient do not usually require such cover, and it is sufficient to maintain as sterile a surgical environment as possible.

The patient must be warned of possible postoperative sequelae. Bleeding is rarely a problem but if it does occur pressure should be applied to the wound with a damp linen pad, as an emergency measure before help is sought. The patient should also be advised to return to the surgery if the pain becomes intolerable; if soft tissue swelling progresses to the extent that the eye closes or swallowing proves painful or difficult; or if he or she feels toxic rather than simply discomforted.

Despite the possible hazards, postoperative recovery is usually uneventful.

Chapter 9

Operative Technique: Treatment of Specific Teeth

Upper Anterior Teeth 321 | 123

Upper central incisor

The treatment of this tooth seldom causes problems.

Upper lateral incisor

The root of the upper lateral incisor is usually retroclined and may be tilted laterally if the arch is crowded. As a result the apex may be deeply placed in the alveolar bone and in such circumstances can more easily be located if the initial identification of the root-face is made relatively coronally.

The angle at which the root lies means that access to the apical canal will usually be very restricted unless the root-tip is resected at an acute angle. The resection must be started sufficiently far down the root-face to ensure that the complete root-tip, including the apical foramen, is removed (Figure 9.1). The root canal is often elongated in cross-section, requiring to be sealed with a retrograde amalgam.

Upper canine

The prominent upper canine root is usually easily identified and apicected. The canine eminence may

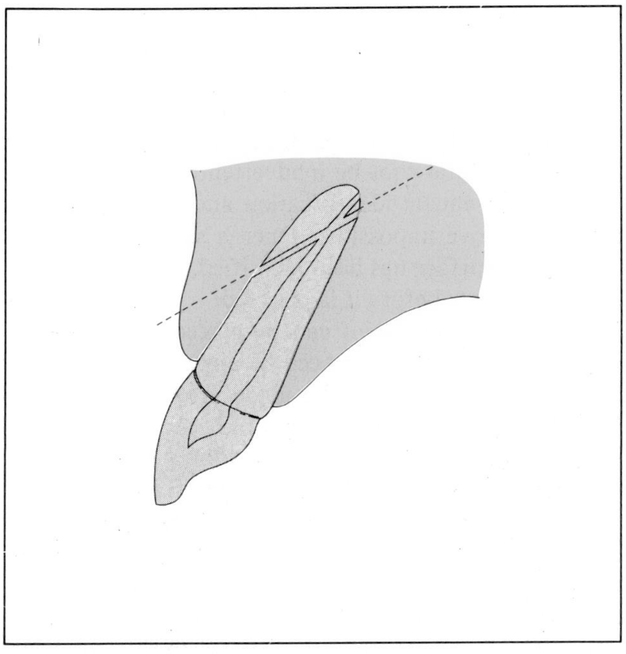

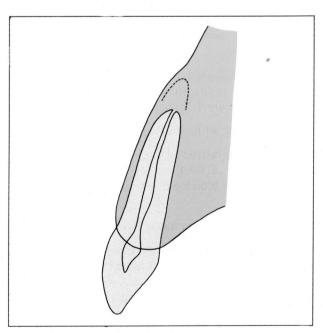

Figure 9.1 *Upper lateral incisor. The apex is often deeply placed and an acutely angled resection is required for access. A palatally placed apical foramen may otherwise be missed*

Figure 9.2 *Upper canine. The canine eminence may sometimes fail to reflect the position of the underlying root-tip, which must be exposed at a more coronal level*

occasionally fail exactly to reflect the position of the underlying root which terminates, and must be exposed, at a slightly more coronal level (Figure 9.2).

Access to the apex may be restricted by the buccal reflection if the root is particularly long. A miniature handpiece head is useful in this situation.

Upper Posterior Teeth (7654 | 4567)

The maxillary antrum

Many dentists are deterred from attempting an apicectomy when radiographs show the root of a tooth to be closely related to the maxillary antrum (Figures 9.9 and 9.10). The palatal root apex can usually be reached only by means of a trans-antral approach. In my opinion, such treatment is the province of the oral surgeon, not the restorative dentist.

The buccal roots of upper posterior teeth can nearly always be treated surgically without risk. Careful bone removal will usually allow the apices to be isolated without involvement of the antral cavity, or at worst with the exposure of small areas of unperforated antral lining. The risk of antral exposure can further be reduced by drilling the buccal bone and approaching the root from in front and below, *never from above* (Figure 9.3a).

The isolated root apex often lies adjacent to the antrum, separated on occasions only by a thickness of mucosal lining. There is always a risk that the resected tip may be displaced either into the antral cavity or beneath its lining. This cannot happen if the apical part of the root is burred down to the desired level, rather than resected (Figure 9.3b).

Small antral perforations are of no consequence provided:

(1) A properly designed, adequately sized envelope flap has been cut so that the line of closure lies on sound bone (*see* Figure 7.2e, page 42).

(2) Postoperative antibiotics are prescribed.

(3) The patient is instructed to avoid raising intra-antral pressure (for a week or so) as, for example, by vigorous nose-blowing or swimming.

Upper first premolar (two-rooted)

The upper first premolar is an extremely difficult tooth to apicect, because of the depth at which the fine palatal root is placed. This root cannot reasonably be approached from the palatal for two reasons. First, because palatal flaps are time-consuming to raise and the operation is unpleasant for the conscious patient. Second, because the root apex is situated at or near the level of the hard palate, which prevents the placement of instruments, and thus the preparation and obturation of

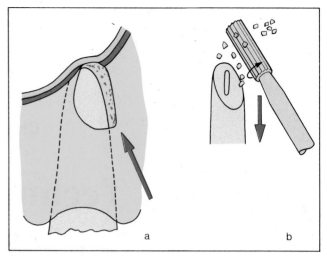

Figure 9.3 *Apicectomy technique for buccal roots in proximity to the antrum.* **a,** *Alveolar bone should be removed from in front of and below the root apex, never from above.* **b,** *The root-tip should be ground down rather than resected in order to avoid the risk of displacement into the antrum. Vision and access are improved by cutting the root surface at a forward and downward angle*

the apical canal (Figure 9.4). Access to the palatal root can usually be gained by way of a buccal approach, provided, first, that the antrum does not extend down between the buccal and palatal roots and, second, that the tooth is not rotated so that its palatal root lies tucked behind the canine.

The buccal root is superficially placed and easily exposed. It is normally necessary to resect a greater length than is usual for other teeth, in order to allow sufficient access to the palatal root (Figure 9.4a). Inter-radicular bone should be drilled away until a small part of the palatal root surface is just revealed (Figure 9.4b). This must be done with great care, for should the palatal root be inadvertently drilled into or through, subsequent identification and isolation of the apex may prove impossible. Once a small part of the palatal root surface has been identified, the apex should be sculpted out, before it is resected.

If an orthograde point can be placed, only a small length of the palatal root need be apicected. However, an oblique resection must be made in order to present the cut root-face and root canal at a convenient angle for the placement of a retrograde filling (Figure 9.4c). Even when a standard bur is used in a childrens-head handpiece it will often be found impossible to approach the apical canal at the correct angle for cavity preparation until an additional wedge of bone has been cut away from above the root-tip (Figures 9.4c and 9.5).

It is sometimes possible to root-fill the palatal root conventionally, the buccal root alone requiring surgical intervention. A combined approach such as this is to be preferred.

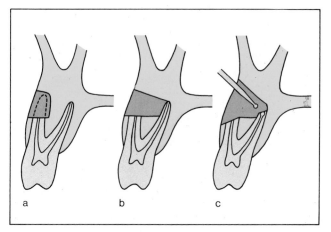

Figure 9.4 *Apicectomy technique used for two-rooted upper premolars.* **a,** *Exposure and resection of the buccal root is made at a relatively coronal level.* **b,** *Inter-radicular bone is removed to identify the palatal root-tip.* **c,** *The palatal root-tip is resected obliquely and if necessary an apical cavity is cut. Apically placed bone may have to be removed in order to allow placement of the drill*

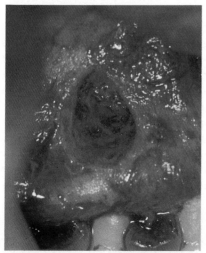

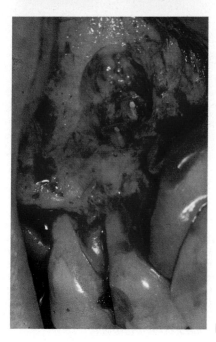

a

b

Upper second premolar

The upper second premolar is usually single-rooted, and thus potentially easy to treat. Its morphology can, however, vary considerably, as may that of the first premolar· (Figures 9.6 and 9.7). When the tooth is single-rooted the resection must be made obliquely; removing a sufficient length of root-tip, so as to ensure either that the ribbon-shaped single canal has completely been exposed, or that any additional palatally placed canal has been identified (Figure 9.7, and *see* Figure 14.2, page 96). If the cut root-tip is of particularly small diameter, the indication is that a second root remains to be identified. Bone loss, softening of the inter-radicular bone, or a sinus extending palatal to the resected root all suggest the presence of a second root. If you are still in doubt, take a radiograph. Now that the superimposed buccal root-tip has been removed, a more deeply placed root should be seen.

When two canals lie closely adjacent in a single root, it is best to run out and fill with amalgam the narrow dentine bridge that lies between them. In this way failure as the result of an unrecognized fissure can be avoided. Similarly, narrow fissures that have been identified,· should be widened sufficiently to allow the amalgam to be placed and properly condensed (Figure 9.6e and f).

Access is made easier if the cut root-face is angled downwards and forwards (*see* Figure 6.5c, page 37).

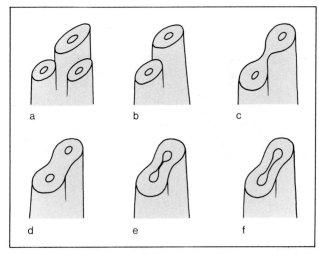

Figure 9.6 *Morphology of apicected upper premolar roots. When root canals are closely placed* **(e)** *the intervening dentine bridge should be run-out and filled, lest microscopic fissures remain unsealed*

Figure 9.5 a, b, *Apicectomy of upper first premolars. A considerable amount of alveolar bone has to be removed in order to gain access to the apex of the palatal root; even when an orthograde technique is used* **(b)**

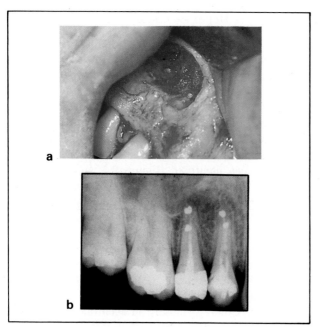

Figures 9.7 a, b, *Apicectomy* 54]. *Note that* 4] *is single-rooted;* 5] *has two roots*

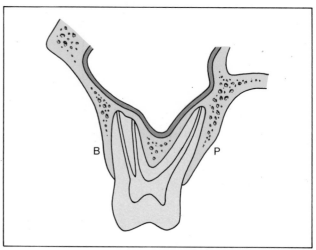

Figure 9.8 *Buccopalatal cross-section of upper first molar region. Note that the two mesiobuccal root canals may terminate at different levels. The antrum hinders access from the buccal to the deeply placed palatal root*

Upper first molar

The palatal root of an upper molar cannot readily be treated surgically. The constraints against a palatal approach have been discussed. A buccal, transalveolar approach is contraindicated for two reasons. First, because the palatal root is so deeply placed that instrumentation would be very difficult. Second, because the antrum is usually interposed and likely to be widely broached (Figure 9.8). Fortunately, palatal root canals are relatively wide and straight and thus amenable to root filling by conventional means. It is usually the buccal roots of upper molars that require surgical intervention and *this should be undertaken only when the palatal root has been satisfactorily obturated with an orthograde filling point* (Figures 9.9c and 9.10c).

The upper lengths of the buccal roots are usually superficially placed and quite accessible (Figure 9.10a, b). However, if the roots are very curved the initial identification should be made relatively coronally, chasing up to the apex (Figure 9.9a,b). The mesiobuccal root

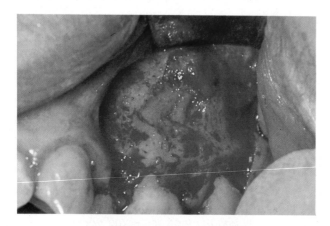

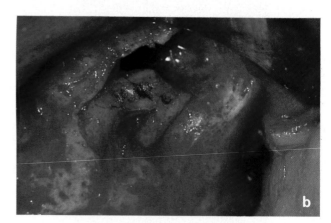

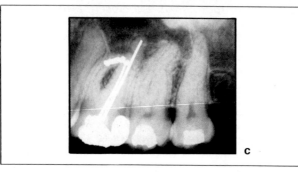

Figure 9.9 *Apicectomy of upper first molar.* **a,** *The superficially placed buccal roots are readily exposed.* **b,** *Resection of the mesiobuccal root has been made at a sufficiently low level to expose a ribbon-shaped canal, which has been run-out and filled.* **c,** *Radiograph taken 6 months postoperatively. The apical lesion has filled in well. Note that the palatal canal has been filled conventionally*

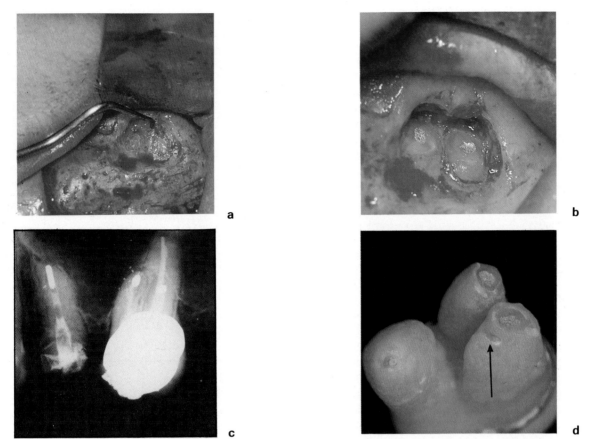

Figure 9.10 *Apicectomy of upper first molar.* **a,** *The apices of the buccal roots are superficially placed and readily exposed.* **b,** *The completed retrograde amalgams (unburnished).* **c,** *Radiograph taken immediately postoperatively. There is a fine scatter of amalgam around the apex of the mesiobuccal root. Note that the* 5| *and the palatal root of* 6| *have been filled conventionally.* **d,** *The case illustrated in parts* **a, b, c** *was referred for treatment in an attempt to cure facial pain of obscure origin. The pain failed to resolve following treatment and the tooth was extracted 6 months postoperatively. The pain continued after extraction. Examination of the tooth* **(d)** *shows the mesiobuccal root to have been resected at too high a level, a palatally placed root canal remaining unidentified and unfilled. The unidentified canal was not the cause of the patient's pain, nevertheless long-term failure might have resulted as a consequence, had the tooth been retained*

is wide buccopalatally, usually having either a single ribbon-shaped canal or two circular canals.

It is usually necessary to place a retrograde amalgam seal in the mesiobuccal root because of the irregular cross-section of the canals (Figure 9.9b,c). Care must be taken not to make the resection at too high a level lest a palatally placed canal remains undetected and unfilled (Figures 9.8 and 9.10d). An orthograde point can sometimes satisfactorily be cemented into the circular distal root canal once the apex has been resected.

Upper second molar

The apices of the buccal roots are often deeply placed beneath the lowermost part of the zygomatic buttress and it is thus best to make the initial identification of the root-face at a relatively coronal level (Figure 9.11). There is usually a single circular root canal in each root and orthograde or retrograde obturation techniques may be used, as appropriate.

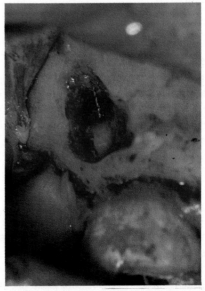

Figure 9.11 *Apicectomy of distal root upper second molar. The root apex was deeply placed and the root was therefore exposed at a relatively coronal level. The canal is being instrumented, prior to obturation by means of an orthograde + retrograde technique*

Lower Teeth

Flap reflection

Envelope flaps should routinely be cut in the lower jaw. The mentalis and buccinator muscles are attached at a relatively high level along the body of the mandible and although the periosteum can be released to any depth, the flap itself can seldom be reflected to the level of the root apices. Thus, the operating site tends to lie within a tissue pouch, with the result that vision and access are impeded. This is not a problem in the upper jaw where the muscle attachments are usually above the level of the root apices.

The mental nerve

The mental nerve usually emerges from its foramen below and between the roots of the lower first and second premolars (*see* Figure 9.16). Vertical relieving incisions are best not cut in this area but, if unavoidable, they should be made short.

When canine or premolar teeth are to be treated, the position of the mental foramen should be determined preoperatively by means of periapical and OPG radiographs. During flap reflection the periosteum should be carefully released to a level below the root apices, such that the operator may ensure either that the mental nerve cannot be seen and is thus not subject to risk; or that the mental foramen and nerve are just visible and can be avoided thereafter. Occasionally, it may prove impossible to distinguish between the mental nerve and an epithelialized sinus arising from an apical lesion. If there is the slightest risk that the nerve may be damaged it is best to abandon the apicectomy. A lost tooth can be replaced prosthetically; mental anaesthesia is likely to be permanent.

Bleeding

Block injections must be supplemented with infiltrations, placed buccal and lingual to the operating site, of a local anaesthetic solution containing a vasoconstrictive agent. Despite this, bleeding can be troublesome during surgery on the lower jaw because the thick alveolar plate hampers diffusion of the anaesthetic solution.

Lower incisors

The ends of the lower incisor roots are usually placed deeply beneath the bone that forms the upper part of the chin. This, plus the problems of flap resection, discussed earlier, results in impeded vision of and access to the root apex. In order to overcome these problems it is necessary to resect the root-tip at an acute angle. Unless the operator is careful he may fail, either completely to expose a ribbon-shaped canal, or to identify a second, lingually placed canal.

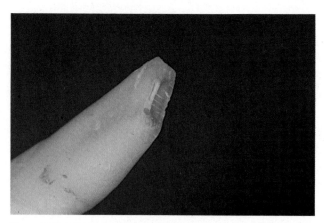

Figure 9.12 *Lower central incisor. The root canal, exposed by resection of the root-tip, is narrow and elongated in cross-section and can satisfactorily be sealed only with a retrograde amalgam filling*

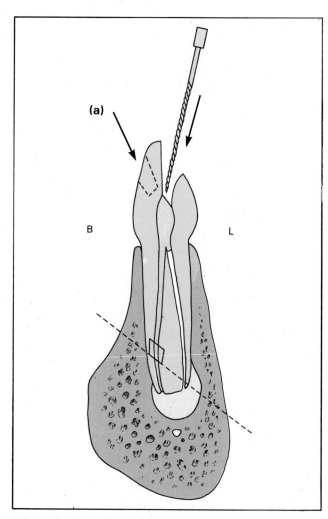

Figure 9.13 *Apicectomy lower incisor. Resection of the root-tip may widely expose a previously undiagnosed or unfilled lingual canal. This must be sealed. Note access and path of insertion* **(a)**, *necessary to instrument the lingual canal*

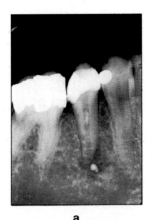

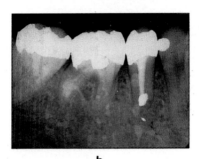

a

b

Figure 9.14 *Apicectomy* $\overline{5|}$. **a**, *Preoperatively.* **b**, *One year postoperatively*

A single root canal exposed following apicectomy is usually long and thin in its cross-section; because of this it can be sealed satisfactorily only by the placement of a retrograde amalgam filling (Figure 9.12). The smallest possible bur must be used to run out the cavity if the narrow root is not to be perforated. Similarly, a very fine plugger, such as a blunted probe, must be employed if the amalgam is to be adequately condensed. Conventional root fillings in lower incisors often fail because only one of two canals has been identified or can be filled (usually the buccal). Attempts to resolve the problem by means of apicectomy will not succeed unless the second, unfilled canal is identified and sealed (Figure 9.13).

It is common practice to root fill lower incisors, prior to raising the flap and resecting the root-tip. This approach is usually doomed to failure because, more often than not, only the buccal canal is identified and filled, with the result that the unfilled lingual canal is widely opened to the tissues following resection of the root-tip (Figure 9.13).

Lower canine

The lower canine root is comparatively long and this further hinders vision and access. In its two-rooted form the tooth is extremely difficult to treat.

Lower premolars

Visibility and access are usually sufficient. The root apices are relatively deeply placed beneath the cortical

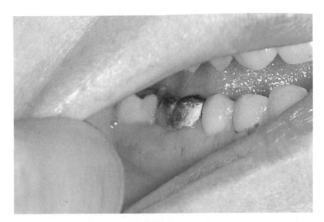

Figure 9.15 *Case illustrated in Figure 9.19, 1 week postoperatively. Note the sufficient access that allowed surgery to be undertaken*

plate, but once exposed may be sealed by means of orthograde or retrograde techniques, as appropriate (Figure 9.14).

Lower first molar

The lower first molar is particularly difficult to treat well by surgical means, principally because access is so very poor. The buccal flap cannot be reflected to the level of the root apices as a consequence of the high muscle attachments; more importantly, the corner of the mouth impedes the placement and manipulation of instruments. In patients with small mouths and tight lips this can prove to be an insurmountable problem. Thus, before making a commitment to apicect it is sensible to assess the degree of access by gently retracting the corner of the patient's mouth. Unless a good depth of alveolus distal to the lower first molar can be exposed (Figure 9.15) the operative difficulties are likely to be severe if not insuperable.

It is usually the narrow, curved canals of the mesial root that require surgical intervention and, whenever possible, a conventional root filling should be placed in the straighter and wider distal canal(s) (Figure 9.18 and *see* Figure 5.17b, page 32).

The lower first molar is more or less centrally placed between the buccal and lingual plates of the mandible and on the buccal side its roots are covered by a considerable thickness of cortical plate and cancellous bone (Figures 9.16 and 9.17). Because of the poor access it is seldom possible to sculpt-out and isolate the root apices and it is usually necessary to identify and expose the root surface some way along its length. An oblique resection is then made with a wide fissure bur, taking care not to penetrate the lingual plate, and the apical portion elevated upwards and outwards (Figures 9.17 and 9.18). The resection can be difficult to do because of the buccolingual breadth of the root. Elevation may also cause problems if, as is often the case, the dentine is brittle.

In most cases it is necessary to insert a retrograde seal, and placement of the amalgam requires dexterity.

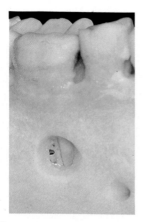

Figure 9.16 *The mental foramen is situated below and between the roots of the first and second premolars. Part of the mesial root of* $\overline{6\,1}$ *has been exposed and is deeply placed beneath a thickness of buccal cortical plate*

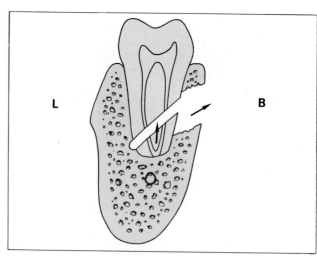

Figure 9.17 *Buccolingual section through lower first molar region. Because of the restricted access it is usually necessary to resect the root obliquely with a relatively wide fissure bur, elevating the lower portion upwards and outwards*

Lower second molar

I have never attempted to apicect this tooth. The roots are deeply placed and the operative problems formidable.

Large Apical Lesions

The presence of a periapical granuloma or dental cyst is seldom a contraindication to apical surgery. Frequently, the enucleation and curettage of such lesions creates working space so that it is relatively easy to reach the apices of roots that would otherwise be inaccessible (*see* Figure 7.2, page 42). This holds true particularly for lower premolar and molar teeth, as illustrated in Figure 9.19.

Problems

The decision whether or not to apicect a particular tooth is a matter of fine clinical judgement. The likely operative difficulties, the importance of the tooth in a treatment plan, and the patient's wishes must all be considered. The operation should not be undertaken unless a successful outcome can reasonably be expected; many teeth, particularly first premolars and lower molars, are not amenable to treatment. Despite careful preoperative assessment, unexpected problems may arise during the operation and, in these circumstances, good dentistry is often best served by extracting the tooth (immediately or at a later appointment) rather than by fruitlessly destroying tissue. If you are inexperienced in surgical endodontic techniques, it is perhaps sensible to pace the development of your surgical skills. First, gain experience on upper anterior

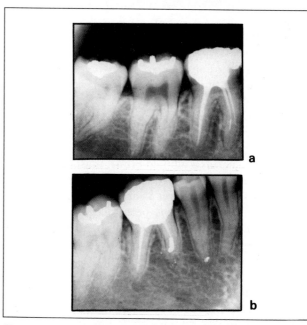

Figure 9.18 *Apicectomy of lower first molar.* **a,** *Preoperative radiograph.* **b,** *Radiograph taken 3 years postoperatively. Note the length of mesial root resected and the oblique resection that was required in order to obtain access*

teeth, progress to upper first molars, then to upper premolars and lower incisors. I would suggest that lower molars and premolars should be attempted only when considerable confidence and expertise has been developed. It is no disgrace to refer; rather, the willingness to acknowledge ones' limitations is a mark of clinical maturity (and in the current climate of litigation, of commonsense!).

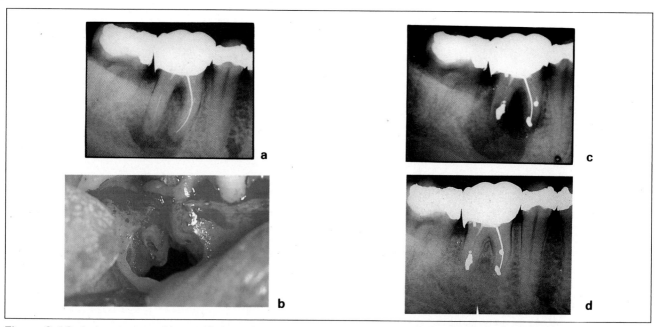

Figure 9.19 *Apicectomy of lower first molar.* **a,** *Radiograph taken 4 months preoperatively.* **b,** *The roots have been exposed following the removal of buccal plate and curettage of pathological soft tissues. No curettage was made at the depth of the lesion in order to avoid damaging the inferior dental nerve.* **c,** *Radiograph taken immediately postoperatively.* **d,** *Radiograph taken 2 years postoperatively. There has been a complete infilling of bone. Clinically the tooth is firm and symptomless. The patient had been referred to her practitioner for the removal of the distal overhang*

Chapter 10

Operative Technique: Fractured Posts and Instruments

Reamers, files or posts that have fractured at the coronal end of the root canal should if possible be withdrawn coronally. Many techniques have been described (Figure 10.1), including the use of fine burs, fine forceps, endodontic instruments and tapped threads. The Masseran trephine is particularly effective (Figure 10.2). Broken spiral lentulae are difficult to remove, especially when they have jammed and broken whilst being rotated by a dental engine. It is not commonly realized that a spiral lentula is withdrawn from a canal by twisting in the direction that it is normally used, i.e. clockwise.

The use of ultrasonically or subsonically activated endodontic instruments is increasingly and effectively being used to dislodge obstructions from within root canals. Nevertheless, such non-invasive methods will occasionally fail, and recourse must be made to surgical intervention.

Fractured Instrument lying wholly within the Apical Part of the Root Canal

If a small length of broken instrument lies within the apical part of a root it may be removed *in situ*, within a length of resected root (Figure 10.3). However, if it is

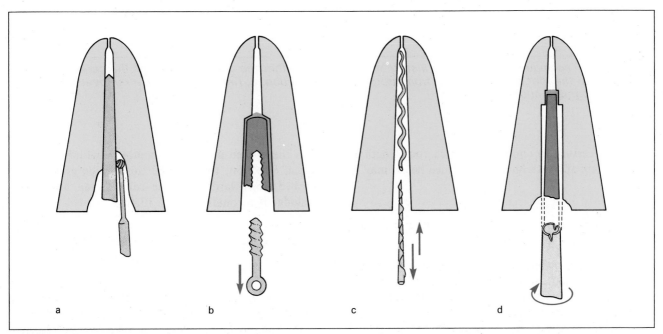

Figure 10.1 *Means of removing fractured instruments and posts coronally.* **a,** *Long-shanked round bur. Exposed post grasped with fine forceps.* **b,** *Tapped thread; bulky, soft metal only.* **c,** *Manipulation with file or reamer.* **d,** *Masseran trephine*

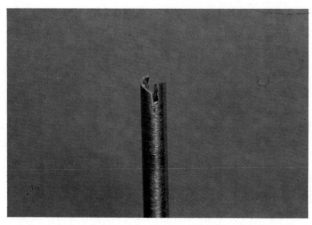

Figure 10.2 *Masseran trephine, used to cut a channel in the dentine, from around the obstruction*

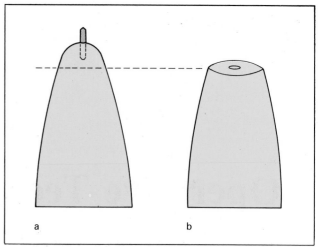

Figure 10.3 *A small, apically retained fragment may be removed within the resected root-tip*

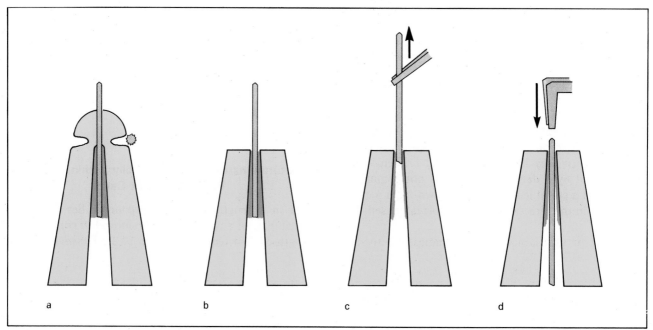

Figure 10.4 *Techniques for removing instruments retained within the greater length of the canal.* **a, b,** *The apical part of the root is ground away from around the obstruction.* **c,** *Retained fragment removed apically.* **d,** *Retained fragment pushed coronally*

deemed necessary to conserve as much root length as possible, one of the techniques described below may be tried.

Fractured Instrument lying within the Greater Length of the Root Canal

Most broken instruments will have jammed in the narrow, apical part of the root canal. If the apical part of the root is carefully burred away, the end of the fractured instrument may sometimes be grasped and withdrawn apically from the wider coronal length of root canal in which it is no longer impacted (Figures 10.4 and 10.5).

If the broken instrument cannot be withdrawn in an apical direction, the exposed tip may be grasped and pushed downwards into the canal in an attempt to dislodge it coronally (Figure 10.4d).

Fractured Instrument lying within the Middle Length of the Root Canal

A coronal withdrawal is necessary either if the instrument lies within the mid-length of the root canal and cannot be exposed as the result of an apical resection, or if the end of the instrument is inadvertently resected, together with the root-tip. Apical resection and the concomitant removal of adjacent bone should create

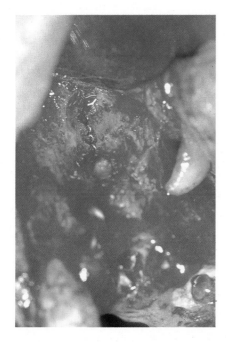

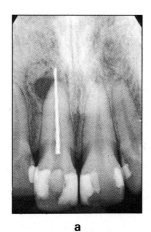
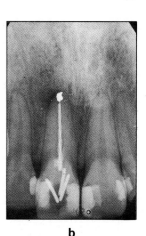

a   b

Figure 10.7 *Fractured reamer treated incorrectly by means of apicectomy. Healing is incomplete at the 6-month review (**b**) and this, plus the difficulty in placing a post and core, emphasizes the desirability of attempting to remove the obstruction by way of the crown*

Figure 10.5 *Fractured spiral lentula exposed by dissection of the root-tip and ready to be released*

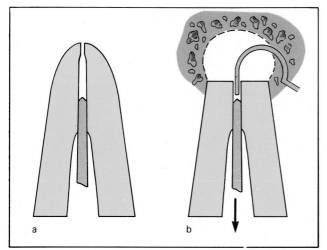

Figure 10.6 *Technique for removing instruments retained in the mid-length of the root canal. **b,** Resection of the apical tip allows a probe to be placed and a dislodging force applied*

enough access to allow an instrument, such as a blunted sickle probe, to be pushed down the root canal, hopefully so as to dislodge the obstruction in a coronal direction (Figure 10.6).

Irremovable Obstructions

A fractured instrument or post may rarely remain inextricably jammed within the canal. It is usually necessary in such cases to place an apical amalgam seal (Figure 10.7). This may require the drilling away of a small length of the obstruction, in order to create an apical cavity. Endodontic instruments and preformed posts are particularly difficult to deal with in this manner and require the frequent replacement of steel burs, or the use of tungsten carbide burs. The Kavo apicectomy handpiece may be used, or a high speed conventional handpiece with tungsten carbide or diamond burs. Subsequent restoration of the tooth crown may be problematical if a fractured instrument is left within the root canal. (*See* Restoration of the Apicected Tooth, Chapter 13.)

Chapter 11

Operative Technique: Repair of Perforations; Replantation

'Apicectomy' approach

Root perforation can result from internal or external resorption (Figure 11.1). The commonest cause is iatrogenic damage as a result of incorrect instrumentation during endodontic treatment, or more usually, the subsequent preparation of a post hole.

A perforation cannot satisfactorily be repaired by cementing a post into the perforation channel. Cement is displaced into the periodontal tissues as the post is seated. The imperfect adaptation of a casting results in the exposure of large amounts of cement lute; and the post can seldom be prepared so as to terminate flush with the root-face (Figures 11.2 and 11.9). The same constraints preclude the use of cast posts, to form the definitive apical seal in either conventional endodontic or apicectomy procedures. If a post is to be cemented at the time of apicectomy, it should be constructed so as to be slightly shorter than the root canal, the seal being made secure with a retrograde filling.

Attempts can be made to obturate a large perforation with a seal of amalgam placed by way of the root canal; or calcium hydroxide can be similarly applied in attempt to promote repair. However, such measures are not always successful and surgery may be required. If a surgical repair is undertaken perforations are usually sealed with silver amalgam, using surgical techniques similar to those described for apicectomy.

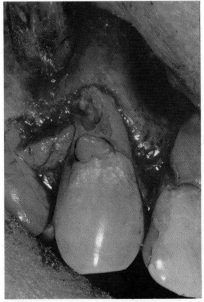
a

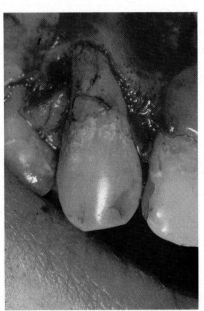
b

Figure 11.1 a, *Idiopathic low-level resorption on the buccal surface of the root of 3| . (b), Repair of perforation with an amalgam seal. The flap was replaced to its original level. The buccal, soft-tissue periodontal pocket was not eliminated*

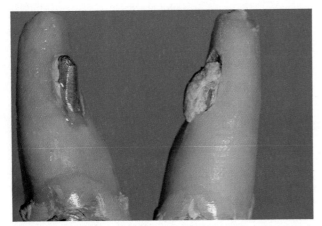

Figure 11.2 *Palatal perforations* 1|1. *Note the size of the perforations caused by the oblique angle of penetration and also partly by resorption of the dentine. The fit of the posts is poor and an excess of cement has been forced into the tissues (referred). The case would have been amenable to elective replantation*

Diagnosis

The creation of a perforation is usually accompanied by pain, and the mishap is thus immediately apparent to both dentist and patient. The location of the perforation can often by determined by carefully probing the canal walls with a file or reamer. This will demonstrate a sensitive area, which is distinctively spongy and tacky to the touch. The instrumentation will, in addition, usually initiate bleeding of greater vigour than would be expected from a simple broaching of the apical constriction. The use of an endosonic apex locator may also be of value in the identification of a root perforation.

Large perforations in the mesial or distal wall of the root can usually be seen on radiographs, but buccal or palatal perforations are difficult to identify and impossible to distinguish by these means.

The orientation of a perforated post, and thus the location of the perforation, can readily be determined radiographically. Mesial and distal perforations are immediately apparent (Figures 11.9b and 11.16a) and buccal and palatal perforations can be distinguished by means of the parallax technique illustrated in Figures 11.3 and 11.4. A buccal or palatal root perforation should be suspected when symptoms persist following root treatment or crowning, despite radiographic evidence of a well-placed filling point or post (Figure 11.4a). The perforation can usually be demonstrated by making additional exposures at different angles in the same vertical plane (Figure 11.4b), or by a profile view (*see* Figure 11.21a, page 77).

Prognosis

The repair of perforations is perhaps the least successful of the surgical techniques employed in endodontics and, as such, offers scope for research and development. Access is often inadequate or non-existent, particularly

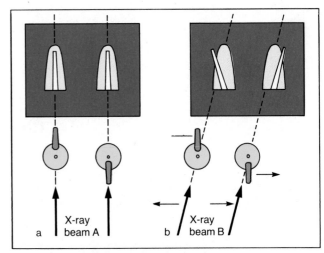

Figure 11.3 *When the X-ray tube is moved mesially or distally a post that has perforated palatally will appear to move in the same direction as the tube. A post that has perforated bucally will appear to move in the opposite direction to the tube*

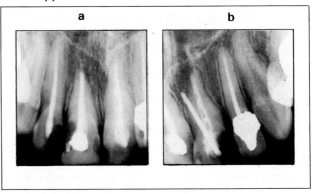

Figure 11.4 a, b, *A palatal perforation of* |1, *demonstrated by the parallax technique illustrated in Figure 11.3. In* **b,** *the tube was angled distally, i.e. towards the left from the right*

when the perforation is situated on the approximal or palatal aspect of the root. In addition, the periodontal tissues may react unfavourably to the large areas of amalgam that have often to be placed. The following factors must be considered:

(1) the location in the root of the perforation:
   (a) aspect (mesial, distal, buccal, palatal)
   (b) level (high, middle, low)

(2) the size of the perforation

(3) the probable age of the perforation.

These factors are interrelated and some, such as the size of the perforation, can be accurately determined only at the time of operation. Thus, perforations cannot be simply classified and each case must be treated according to first principles and practical exigency.

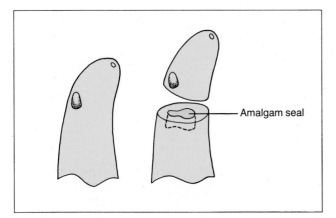

Figure 11.5 *A high-level perforation can be removed by resecting the damaged length of root*

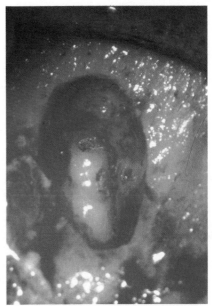

Figure 11.6 *Repair of high-level perforation*

Location of the perforation

Aspect

Perforations on the buccal, buccomesial and buccodistal aspects of the root can usually be reached and repaired. However, such repairs, no matter how perfect technically, will sometimes fail because of other factors, such as the size of the perforation, or the loss of supporting alveolar bone *(see below)*.

Palatally orientated and palatal perforations are difficult to treat because of inadequate access and, in the latter case, the prognosis is usually poor.

Level

High perforations, including those on the palatal, can sometimes be eliminated by resecting the damaged uppermost length of root (Figures 11.5 and 11.17b).

Mid-level perforations, when newly created, can usually be treated successfully provided that access is adequate.

If the perforation is of long standing, chronic infection and the drainage of pus will often have caused the destruction of coronally placed alveolar bone and the consequent formation of a pocket. It is most unlikely that bone will reform following repair of the perforation. On the buccal, a soft tissue attachment can be hoped for, provided, first, that the perforation is sufficiently high and not too large and, second, that the contaminated root-face has been thoroughly planed (Figure 11.7). Interproximal bone loss results in the formation of an irreparable and uncleansable infrabony pocket. The prognosis is thus very poor (Figure 11.8).

Low-level perforations in the mesial or distal wall of the root have a poor prognosis for the reasons that have

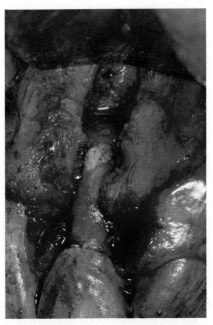

Figure 11.7 *A mid-level buccal perforation. Drainage of pus from the apical lesion has caused the loss of supporting buccal bone. The perforation is sufficiently high to offer hope of a soft tissue attachment to the thoroughly planed root-face*

been discussed above. There is often a severe destruction of tissue (Figure 11.9).

Perforations of the buccal wall can usually be repaired (Figure 11.1), composite resin being used when amalgam is likely to prove unaesthetic. Pocket formation can be reduced either by replacing the flap at a more apical level or, if there is a sufficient height of keratinized tissue, by performing a gingivoplasty. A less

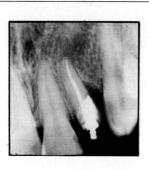

Figure 11.8 *A mid-level interproximal perforation. The perforation has caused the development of an infrabony pocket. Despite an (imperfect) attempt at repair, the prognosis is poor*

unsightly alternative is to replace the flap in its original position, controlling the pocket by the implementation of a high level of oral hygiene. A relatively small and coronally placed perforation can be further exposed by moving the root coronally with orthodontic traction. The exposed perforation can then more easily be repaired; or the damaged root may be resected prior to the construction of a post-retained crown.

Size of perforation

Perforations are often found at operation to be larger than expected. First, because of the oblique angle at which the preparatory instrument has cut through the root (Figures 11.2 and 11.9b); second, because inflammatory tissue can, in longstanding cases, exert an odontoclastic effect, enlarging the original perforation and often saucerizing the adjacent root-face (Figures 11.2 and 11.10).

The bigger the perforation the more difficult it is to place a well-condensed, properly shaped, uncontaminated seal. The prognosis is likely to be further worsened because of the large surface area of amalgam in contact with the tissues.

Age of perforation

Longstanding perforations are likely to be large and associated with irreversible bone loss *(see above)*.

Surgical Procedure

The principles of surgical repair are similar to those described for 'apicectomy'. A flap is raised and the terminal part of the perforation freshened with a round bur to form a cavity into which an amalgam seal is packed. In practice three factors determine the technique to be employed in the repair:

(1) Whether the perforation was identified prior to cementation of the post

(2) Whether the perforation was identified following its cementation

(3) The location of the perforation

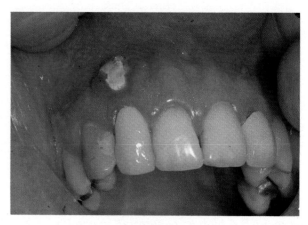

a

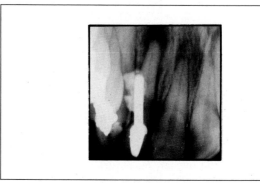

b

Figure 11.9 a, *A low-level buccal perforation. Because of the size of the post and the obliquity of the perforation, a large amount of tissue had been destroyed* **(b)**, *and the tooth was extracted. The patient, a dental nurse, presented with the perforation about 1 year following placement of the post*

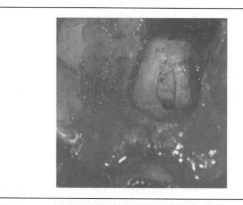

Figure 11.10 *A mid-level perforation. Longstanding infection has resulted in saucerization of the buccal root surface. Care must be taken not to overfill this saucerized area with amalgam. Because a new post was to be constructed at a later date, the underlying root canal was packed with gutta-percha to prevent it being filled with amalgam. Although the perforation is large, the prognosis is fair because coronally placed buccal bone has not been lost*

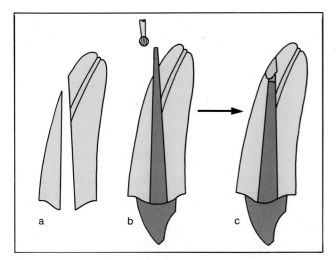

Figure 11.11 *A high-level perforation* **(a)** *may be treated by cementing a shortened post and placing a terminal seal* **(c)***. An established high-level perforation by a cemented post* **(b)** *may be treated by drilling away the post to below the level of the root face, then placing a terminal seal* **(c)**

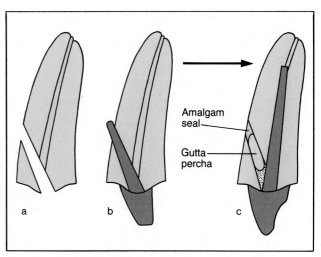

Figure 11.12 *A middle, or low-level perforation* **(a)** *is usually best treated by cutting a correctly positioned post hole and repairing the perforation after the new post has been cemented* **(c)***. Malpositioned perforated posts* **(b)** *should first be extracted*

Identification of perforation prior to cementation of post

If the *apical part* of the root has been perforated, construction of the post may be continued, its length being reduced sufficiently to allow placement of the terminal amalgam seal (Figure 11.11a and c).

When the perforation lies in the *middle or lower* part of the root, a new and correctly placed post hole must be cut to which a new post is constructed (Figure 11.12a and c; Figure 11.14).

In both cases it is best to cement the post at the time of operation, just prior to preparing and sealing the perforation. Very occasionally, it may be necessary to repair a perforation prior to the construction and cementation of a post and core. In such circumstances that part of the root canal which lies beneath the perforation should be obturated with gutta-percha in order both to form a base against which the amalgam is condensed and to prevent the amalgam forming an impassable obstruction within the canal (Figures 11.10 and 11.12c).

Identification of perforation following cementation of post

A long post that has perforated the *apical part* of the root can often be difficult to remove. Rather than risk fracturing the root, it is usually best to drill away enough of the post to allow the placement of an amalgam seal (Figure 11.11b and c).

New steel burs can be used to cut metal but they blunt rapidly and must be replaced frequently; alternatively, tungsten carbide or diamond burs can be used in a high-speed handpiece, cooled with a saline drip. Fine metal filings will often be seen on the postoperative radiograph to have infiltrated into the cancellous bone spaces (see Figure 2.2b, page 15).

A post that has perforated the *middle or lower part* of a root is unlikely to be sufficiently retentive, particularly after it has been cut down to below the level of the root-face. Instead, the post should be extracted and a new post constructed to fit a correctly prepared post hole (Figure 11.12b and c). The new post should be cemented at the time of operation, just prior to repairing the perforation.

Location of the perforation

Buccal perforation

Buccal perforations are usually simple to repair.

Mesial or distal perforation

It is often difficult to obtain adequate access to a mesial or distal perforation, particularly when the lesion is situated towards the palatal.

Greater reach can be obtained, at the expense of fine control, by using an extra-long right-angle bur (Meisinger) in a childrens-head handpiece (Figure 11.13). Apically where the root tapers, and coronally in those cases where the neighbouring root does not lie immediately adjacent, it is sometimes possible to remove sufficient interstitial bone to allow the perforation to be approached directly (Figure 11.14).

The adjacent root is usually likely to be damaged if a direct approach is made. In such cases, access to the perforation can be gained by way of a small channel

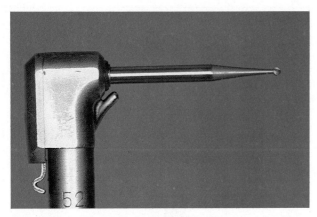

Figure 11.13 *An extra-long right-angle bur used in a standard or childrens-head handpiece will afford extra reach, but at the expense of fine control*

cut in the buccoapproximal aspect of the root (Figures 11.15, 11.16); in effect, preparing a small mesiobuccal or distobuccal cavity.

The blade of a 'flat plastic' instrument can be held against the root surface to form a matrix against which the amalgam is condensed and contoured (Figure 11.18b).

Palatal perforation

Very occasionally, a high palatal perforation can be eliminated by resecting the apical length of root (Figure 11.17b). Alternatively, removal of the post and recementation of a shorter replacement may allow an apicopalatal cavity to be cut and filled by way of an apical approach (Figures 11.17c and 11.18). However, such reclamatory measures are seldom possible.

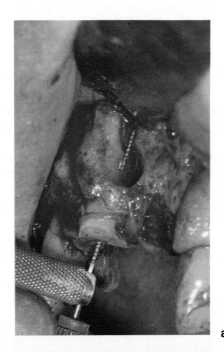

a

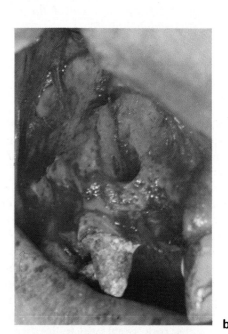

b

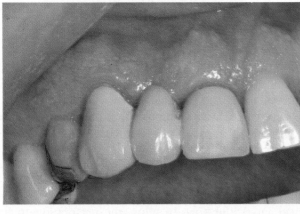

c

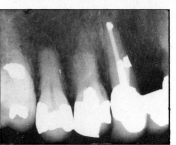

d

Figure 11.14 a, *Repair of a perforation created during the preparation of a post hole for a bridge abutment. The loss of supporting bone, and the lack of an immediately adjacent tooth, allowed a direct approach to be made.* **b,** *The dentist had recut the post hole and supplied a well-fitting, accurately positioned post and core. This was cemented immediately prior to the repair of the perforation and the establishment of an apical seal.* **c,** *The soft tissues 10 months postoperatively.* **d,** *Follow-up radiograph 10 months postoperatively*

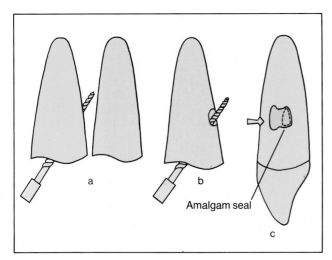

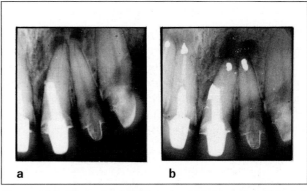

Figure 11.15 *Mid- or low-level interproximal perforations can often not be approached directly because of adjacent roots* (**a**). *Such perforations can be reached indirectly by cutting an access groove in the approximobuccal surface of the root* (**b, c**). *The dotted lines in* (**c**) *indicate the outline of the original perforation*

Figure 11.16 a, b, *Mid-level mesial perforation* ⌐1 *repaired by using the indirect approach. Radiographs taken immediately pre- and postoperatively. Note that the canals have not been filled. This worsens the prognosis*

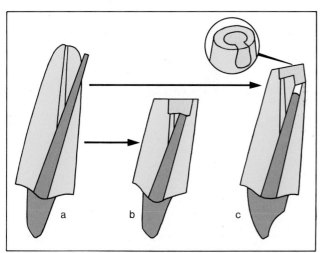

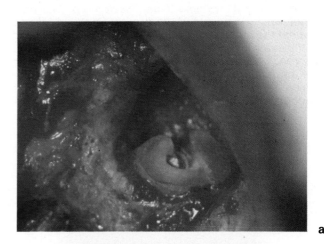

Figure 11.17 *Palatal perforations are extremely difficult to repair. Rarely, the perforation can be resected at the expense of root length* (**b**). *If the post can be shortened* (**c**) *an occlusopalatal repair can occasionally be made* (**see** *Figure 11.18*)

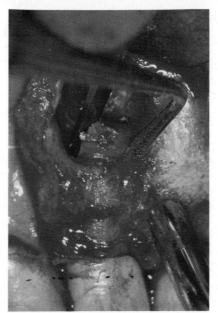

Figure 11.18 a, b, *Distopalatal perforation repaired by cutting and filling an occlusopalatal cavity, approached from the occlusal. Note the use of a 'flat plastic' instrument as a matrix against which to condense and shape the amalgam*

Thermoplasticized gutta-percha

The use of thermoplasticized gutta-percha, delivered by a syringe, offers a way of sealing perforations with gutta-percha applied through the access cavity in the crown of the tooth. However, it may be necessary to raise a flap in order to place a matrix, such as the blade of a 'flat plastic' instrument, so as to control the flow of the material (Figure 11.19).

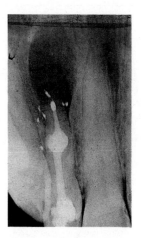

a

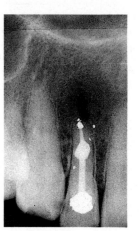

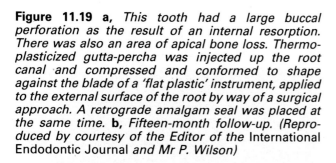

Figure 11.19 a, *This tooth had a large buccal perforation as the result of an internal resorption. There was also an area of apical bone loss. Thermoplasticized gutta-percha was injected up the root canal and compressed and conformed to shape against the blade of a 'flat plastic' instrument, applied to the external surface of the root by way of a surgical approach. A retrograde amalgam seal was placed at the same time.* **b,** *Fifteen-month follow-up. (Reproduced by courtesy of the Editor of the* International Endodontic Journal *and Mr P. Wilson)*

b

Repair of perforations using a replantation technique
A.F. Carmichael and I.E. Barnes

In the authors' experience, except in the most exceptional circumstances where the defect is apically placed, palatal perforations are impossible to repair by conventional surgical methods. The problem can, however, often be overcome by extracting the tooth, repairing the perforation and replanting. The suggestion that such treatment be done is often viewed askance by the patient and the procedure is done with trepidation by the dentist. However, such reservations are misplaced. After all, non-elective replantation works well with the child and the chances of success should increase when the procedure is elective. Of advantage over the avulsed tooth is the fact that the extracted tooth may be kept moistened with saline during the brief period that it is out of the mouth. Of disadvantage is the fact that the tooth must be extracted with forceps, at risk of fracturing a root that has been weakened by the post hole preparation. The avulsed tooth is normally knocked out intact.

In terms of discomfort, patients who have had both an apicectomy and a replantation usually say that the elective replantation is the less traumatic.

Diagnosis

A root perforation may be suspected for the reasons detailed earlier in this chapter. The most usual presentation is a mucosal sinus, and the appearance on periapical radiographs of a bone rarefaction or thickening of the periodontal space on the mesial or distal aspect of a post-filled root – usually some distance from the apex, giving a slight 'spare tyre' effect (Figure 11.20).

Often an initial exploratory operation will be undertaken, for despite the success of the elective replantation, it takes a confident operator to extract a suspect tooth simply on the basis of parallax radiographs or a 'hunch' that the perforation is so palatally placed as to be unreachable by conventional means. This exploratory procedure may afford the opportunity to clear debris and granulations from around the root

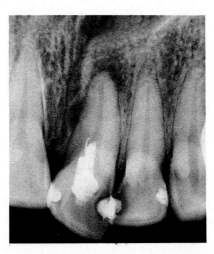

Figure 11.20 *'Spare-tyre' effect of periradicular bone loss, typically seen with root perforation*

(*see* Figure 11.22a). Profile view radiographs which can conveniently be made with standard apical films are perhaps the most reliable guide, but if there are several post crowns in the upper incisor region, the profusion of posts and root canal fillings may confuse the situation (Figure 11.21).

'Planned Extraction and Replantation' (the PEAR technique) should be regarded as the last resort before extracting the tooth and replacing it with a denture or bridge. The technique can also be used to deal with other problems such as dens-in-dente which cannot be dealt with conventionally.

Planning

The proposed PEAR technique must be explained carefully to the patient, in that it is a last resort and does present the risk of failure. The artificial crown may fracture during extraction; or the post may be inadvertently withdrawn – increasing the likelihood of fracturing the hollow, weakened root during the subsequent extraction procedure; or the operator may discover that the root is already split, making further conservative treatment impossible.

The patient should be advised that after the replantation has been carried out, the prognosis is good in the short term. The long-term prognosis, beyond 2 or 3 years, is also good, though root resorption and/or ankylosis may occur.

Technique (*see* Figure 11.22 a–i)

Preparation

If an apicectomy or exploratory operation has been done, it is wise to allow a period of time for the soft and

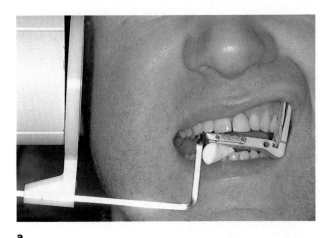

a

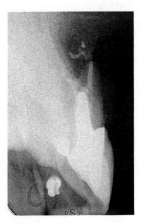

b

Figure 11.21 a, *Technique for taking a profile view of an anterior tooth, using standard periapical film.* **b,** *Profile view of upper central incisor, showing a post that has perforated the palatal aspect of the root. Both cases of Mr A. Carmichael*

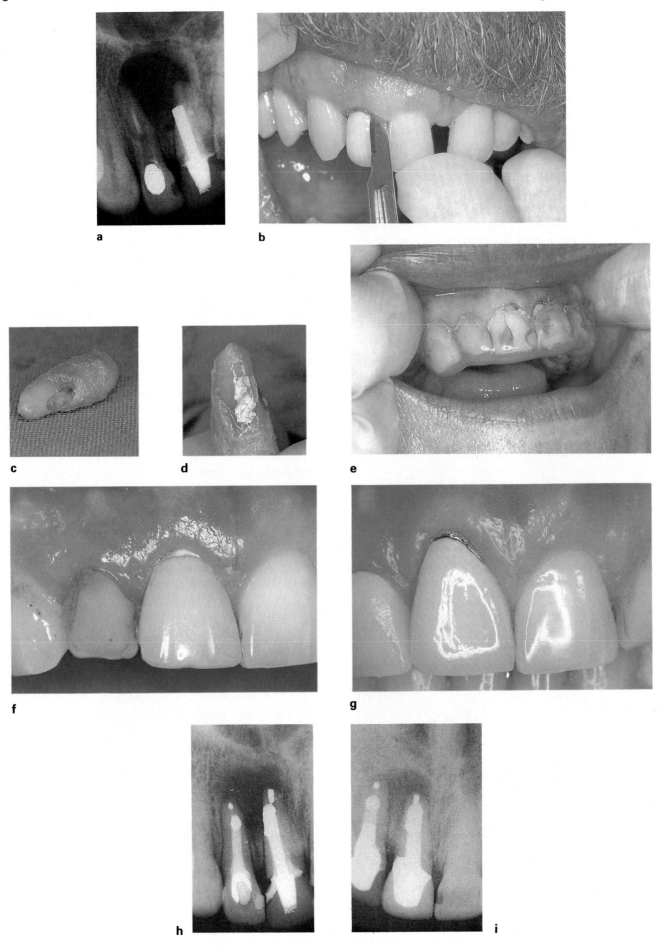

bony tissues to heal and regenerate before undertaking the PEAR technique.

The first stage in the PEAR technique is the taking of an impression of the arch. The model thus produced may be used to construct a soft vinyl splint (Drufomat) and also to prepare an immediate partial denture to be used should the tooth be hopelessly damaged during the extraction. The soft splint also has the advantage that it may be used as a template for the construction of a temporary plastic crown, immediately postoperatively, should the original crown break during the extraction.

The incidence of ankylosis is reduced if a tooth is splinted for as little time as possible – and a week is more than sufficient. A soft splint covering all the teeth in the arch, but not involving the palate, is simple and cheap to prepare. It is simply inserted after the operation, and the sensible patient can be trusted to gently remove it after a day or two, so as to aid in hygiene regimens. Also, it may be that the lack of rigidity helps to prevent the development of ankylosis.

It is probably sensible to give antibiotic cover 1 hour preoperatively (*see* below). At operation the minimal effective increment of anaesthetic is delivered, buccally and palatally or lingually. Dry socket is to be avoided.

Extraction

Extraction may be made easier by first cutting the marginal circular fibres of the periodontal membrane with a knife (Figure 11.22b). If a porcelain crown is present, the forceps should have curved beaks which will grasp the cervical part of the root without contacting the porcelain, as pressure on the crown will cause it to split. Such a technique also serves to prevent the post from being withdrawn, thus weakening the root and increasing the likelihood of root fracture during the extraction. However, care must be taken not to drive the beaks up the periodontal membrane, which at all times should be protected. The extraction should be positive and well controlled. When possible, rotational rather than buccolingual or buccopalatal movements are to be preferred. If to and fro movements are necessary they should be limited in number and firm in execution. Paradoxically, too prolonged and 'gentle' an extraction technique may result in the periodontal membrane being crushed and the root-face burnished. Too vigorous an extraction may break the root or unnecessarily expand the socket.

Repair

As soon as the tooth has been extracted it should be examined to identify the perforation and any projecting post (Figure 11.22c). It is always pleasant to confirm that your diagnosis is correct and the extraction justified. Once this hurdle has been overcome it is possible to proceed with a relative lightness of heart.

It is important not to damage the torn periodontal membrane either by pressure or desiccation. If the tooth has been extracted intact the crown may be held. If the crown and post have been removed during the extraction, it may be necessary to hold the root (vertically between apex and the 'occlusal' root-face, if possible) very gently between the gloved fingers, or in saline soaked gauze. Purpose-made jigs to gently hold the root have been developed (Carmichael).

Immediately upon extraction, the tooth or the root are immersed in sterile physiological saline while the operator examines the socket to ensure that the gum margin has not been lacerated. If there has been no prior exploratory operation, the area of infection which has been identified on the radiograph can be very carefully curetted in order to remove any infected tissue or any excess cement that may have been extruded into the tissues. However, in the absence of excess cement it is doubtful if it is necessary to curette the tissues, and such curettage if done at all should be done circumspectly and only in the immediate area of the lesion.

The root must be kept moist at all times, being immersed frequently in the sterile saline, and the periodontal tissues adhering to its surface must not be traumatized. If the root perforation is open, its margin may be gently freshened with a bur in order to remove grossly stained or softened dentine. However, the deficiency must be kept as small as possible. The same bur may be used to debride within the perforation to remove soft or necrotic tissue. If the metal post projects from the perforation it must be reduced and countersunk to a depth of about 2 mm. This may be done with sterile tungsten carbide or diamond burs in an airotor

Figure 11.22 a, *Large palatal perforation 1|. An exploratory operation was done 2 months prior to replantation, at which time seals were placed apically in 21| and debris and granulations removed.* **b,** *Periodontal fibres cut prior to the extraction (different case from series 11.22c–i).* **c,** *Extracted tooth, showing the palatal perforation. Note, the gauze on which the tooth is resting for photographic purposes is not as wet as it should be.* **d,** *The repaired perforation.* **e,** *The soft splint in place, immediately postoperatively.* **f,** *The tooth in situ 1 week postoperatively.* **g,** *The tooth in situ 19 months postoperatively. There has been some gingival recession. The post is a new one and has been in place for 8 months. It is acid-etch retained to the overprepared, flared canal.* **h,** *Immediate postoperative radiograph.* **i,** *19-month postoperative radiograph. Note, there is an indication of early root resorption. This may be a consequence of the extraction, the replantation, or of the etch technique that was used to retain the new post. The patient has been advised that the prognosis is uncertain at this stage*

run without the system water spray, but in *very* short bursts, the tooth being constantly dipped in the saline so that the temperature does not build up. It must be stressed once again that it is not sufficient merely to cut the post flush with the root-face – this will not effect a seal. The cavity must be sealed with amalgam. The prepared cavity is first cleansed by irrigation with saline under pressure, and is dried with paper points before being filled with amalgam applied with an amalgam gun. Spherical alloy is best used, being patted into position and contour, endeavouring to contaminate as little of the adjacent root surface as possible. Final contouring can be done with the side of a straight probe (Figure 11.22d).

Obturation of canal

The adequacy of the obturation of the apical part of the root canal should have been checked on the preoperative radiographs at the treatment planning stage. Nevertheless, even if the root appears on radiographic examination to be well filled, the adequacy of the apical seal must be assessed visually once the tooth has been extracted. If the apical seal appears to be imperfect, it should be replaced at this time. Similarly, if radiographs have shown a poorly filled length of root canal lying apical to the post, this must be obturated, even though any apical amalgam seal may seem to be sound. If this is not done the debris contained within the canal and the associated tubules can cause postoperative inflammatory resorption of the root. If the canal is to be cleansed it may be necessary to resect an existing apical seal or to resect the root-tip in order to give sufficient access to the files and irrigation needle that are used (for details of the technique see Chapter 7, page 50). The procedure must be done quickly.

In the case of a replanted avulsed tooth, the risk of inflammatory resorption is said to be greatly reduced if antibiotics are prescribed postoperatively. Replantation for the repair of perforations is an elective procedure, and it would seem sensible, therefore, to prescribe antibiotics preoperatively so that the replanted tooth may be inserted into a socket already protected by antibiotic 'cover'.

Replantation

Once the amalgam or amalgams have been smoothed and the root surface checked to ensure that there is no debris adhering to it, the tooth can be reimplanted. The socket should be gently cleansed of blood, using sterile saline applied from a syringe, and the tooth delicately replaced. Once in the socket it is helpful to hold the tooth for some minutes to allow the clotting mechanism to 'tack' the tooth in place.

Splinting

The tooth crown and tissues are then wiped clean and the soft splint placed (Figure 11.22e). Once the tooth has been inserted, analgesics may be prescribed before the anaesthetic wears off. The patient should be instructed in oral hygiene techniques, using mouthwashes (Corsodyl) and cleansing with a soft toothbrush. They may be reassured that the tooth will not fall out when the splint is carefully removed on the day after operation and when the tooth is gently brushed. If the patient is worried, they can return to the surgery on the day after the operation for the initial removal of the splint and the first oral hygiene procedure to be undertaken by the dentist or hygienist. The splint is worn for 7 days after which the patient is reviewed (Figure 11.22f). Another case is illustrated in Figure 11.23.

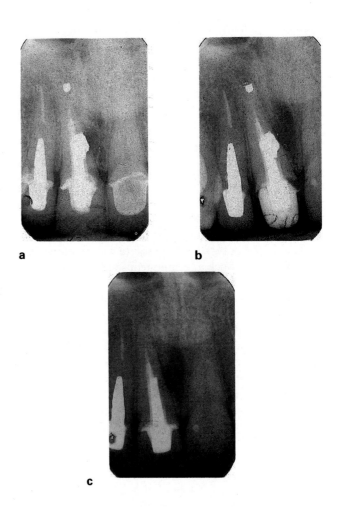

a   b

c

Figure 11.23 a, *Mesio-palatal perforation* 1|. *This was not reparable by way of a conventional approach.* **b,** *Immediately postoperative, following extraction, repair and elective replantation.* **c,** *5-year follow-up. The tooth is firm and symptomless. The radiograph shows a possible slight loss of definition at the end of the root. There is a radiolucent area over the amalgam seal, probably scar or chronic granulation tissue. Case of Mr A. Carmichael*

Root Resorption

Root resorption is likely to be the chief cause of failure following an initially successful replantation. In summary, the following precautions will reduce the risk.

(1) Preoperative antibiotics should be prescribed

(2) The extraction should be atraumatic

(3) The root surface must be kept constantly moist

(4) The root surface must be touched as little as possible

(5) The root canal must be cleansed and filled

(6) The tooth must be replanted quickly

(7) The tooth should be splinted for as short a time as possible.

Chapter 12

Operative Technique: Alternative Methods

Preoperative assessment may indicate that an apicectomy should not be attempted — for example (within the author's competence or incompetence!), when the palatal root of an upper molar requires treatment. Alternatively, insuperable difficulties may unexpectedly arise during the course of the operation itself. Excessive bleeding may occur, it may prove impossible to identify a deeply placed root, or to isolate and resect an apex that is tucked behind an adjacent root. When such problems arise, one course of action is immediately to extract the tooth. However, it is often preferable to suture the flap and allow the wound to heal, following which one of four forms of treatment may be undertaken:

(1) Extraction
(2) Root resection
(3) Tooth hemisection
(4) Replantation.

Detailed consideration of the first three techniques is not appropriate in a basic manual such as this. They are, however briefly dealt with as a pointer to further study. The treatment of root fractures and endodontic implants is also discussed, since both procedures employ surgical techniques that are essentially the same as those described for apicectomy:

(5) Root fracture
(6) Endodontic implants.

Extraction

Extraction, and the provision of a well-made prosthesis, is usually the wisest course of action, if it seems likely that apical surgery will offer merely a small chance of short-term success. When the decision to extract is made during apicectomy, resuturing the flap and allowing a period of healing affords two advantages. First, a well-made temporary prosthesis can be constructed. Second, alveolar bone removed during surgery may reform

above the root, with the result that gingival recession may be less rapid or severe than would be the case were the tooth to be immediately extracted.

Root Resection

If a root can be neither root filled nor apicected it may be resected, provided, first, that the tooth remains sufficiently supported and, second, that the morphology of the treated tooth is compatible with gingival and periodontal health. These constraints usually preclude the treatment by root resection of upper premolars. The palatal roots of upper molars and the mesial or distal roots of lower molars are usually amenable to treatment.

Upper molar: palatal root

The lower part of the palatal root is exposed by the partial reflection of a palatal flap and the removal of alveolar bone. Relieving incisions are best not cut, because of the hazard posed by the palatal artery. Adequate reflection can be achieved by a sufficient extension of the crevicular incision.

It would seem sensible to make the initial root resection with a narrow fissure bur, loosening the retained fragment prior to either judiciously widening the resection and/or removing more palatal bone, in order to allow disimpaction and removal of the root. Following resection, the undersurface of the crown must be contoured to allow cleansing, and the exposed orifice of the pulp chamber should be filled with amalgam which is subsequently polished (Figure 12.1).

Lower molar: mesial or distal root

It is important, before proceeding with the operation, carefully to determine from preoperative radiographs

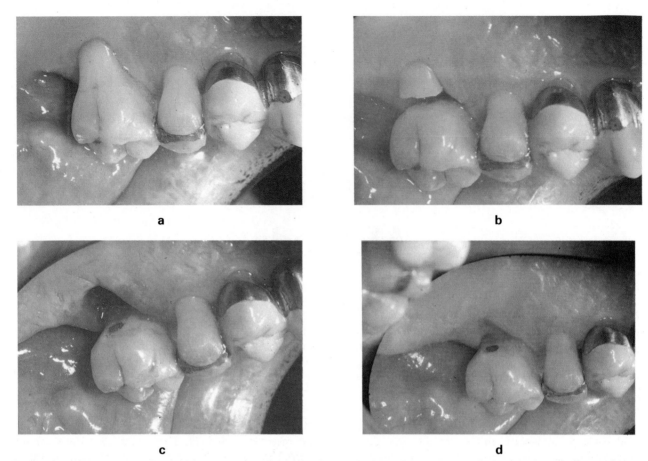

a

b

c

d

Figure 12.1 *Resection of palatal root* 6|, *undertaken for periodontal reasons.* **a,** *Preoperative.* **b,** *Resection cut, made with fissure bur.* **c,** *Immediately following extraction of the root.* **d,** *Early postoperative appearance. Note the cleansible contour of the crown surface, and the polished amalgam seal. (Case reproduced by courtesy of Mr P. Floyd)*

the level of the bifurcation. A low bifurcation precludes resection or hemisection (Figure 12.2). Access is from the buccal. Following resection, the maintenance of adequate levels of cleansing can be difficult, because of the bulbous overhang of the crown (Figure 12.3a). For this reason, hemisection is often the treatment of choice (Figure 12.4).

Hemisection of Lower Molars

Following hemisection of the crown, and removal of the untreatable root, the retained divided crown may be restored with a cast gold restoration, which can be one retainer of a small bridge replacing the lost half tooth (Figure 12.4).

The techniques of resection and hemisection may be further studied from periodontal texts. Treatment for periodontal reasons is not, however, strictly comparable to treatment for endodontic reasons, because the healthy supporting tissues of the non-periodontally involved tooth make release of the resected root more difficult, a problem compounded by the brittleness of the non-vital dentine.

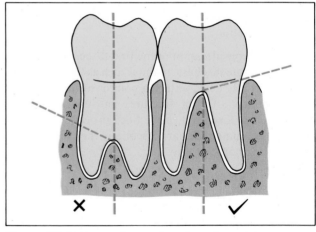

Figure 12.2 *Resection or hemisection of lower molars is possible only if the bifurcation lies at a relatively coronal level*

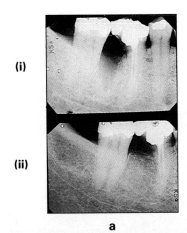

(i)

(ii)

a

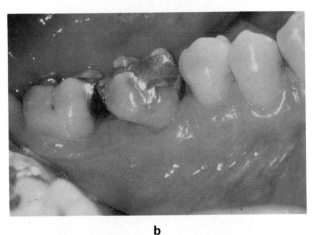

b

***Figure 12.3** **a,** Resection of distal root $\overline{6|}$. (i) Immediately postoperative. (ii) Following bony healing. **b,** Tooth shown in **a,** following bony healing. The gingival health is good, despite the overhang of the crown, which favours plaque accumulation*

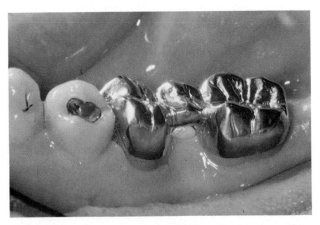

Figure 12.4 *Tooth shown in Figure 12.3b. Hemisection of the crown has allowed a small bridge to be constructed, the retained tooth segment·acting as a mesial abutment. The sanitary pontic allows a high level of cleansing to be maintained. Figures 12.3 and 12.4 illustrate the case of Mr I. Waite, by whose kind permission they are published*

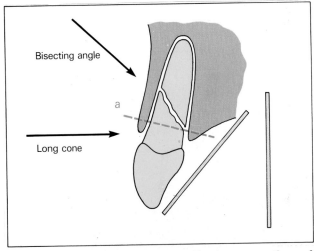

Figure 12.5 *Oblique fracture. Further resection of the root in order to aid visibility and access will unacceptably reduce periodontal support (a). Radiographs taken by the bisecting angle technique may misleadingly show the fracture as a horizontal line. A long-cone technique is preferred*

Replantation

Replantation can be considered when apicectomy proves impossible, in the following circumstances.

(1) When resection or hemisection is not indicated

(2) When close approximation of associated structures such as the mental nerve, maxillary antrum or adjacent roots prevent a surgical approach to the apex

(3) When previous attempts at apicectomy have failed and where it is suspected that a root or root canal remains unidentified

(4) Where a root perforation, inaccessible by other approaches, is to be repaired.

Fractured Roots: Endodontic Implants (Stabilizers)

A detailed consideration of horizontal and oblique root fractures is outside the scope of this book. Such injuries are increasingly being treated either conservatively or by means of conventional endodontic techniques. Occasionally, however, it may be decided to treat such a fracture by removing the apical part of the fractured root and sealing the coronal part. The surgical technique is similar to that described in Chapters 4–7. However, the operation is seldom straightforward. Placement of the seal can be difficult because such fractures seldom extend purely horizontally and frequently run at an angle, downwards and palatally. Vision of, and access to, the root canal are thus severely restricted. It is seldom possible to increase access by levelling or bevelling the end of the retained root because its periodontal support would thus be unacceptably reduced (a, Figure 12.5). An oblique fracture will usually appear on a long cone radiograph as a double line joining at both edges of the root (Figure 12.6). If the X-ray beam runs parallel to an oblique fracture, as in the commonly used bisecting angle technique, the fracture may well appear to be simple and horizontal (Figure 12.5 and Figure 12.7). Unless the dentist is aware of this hazard, the patient may be unduly encouraged as to the prognosis.

Lost periodontal support can be made good by the cementation of an endodontic implant, which extends throughout the length of the socket to wedge slightly into the apical lamina dura. However, such implants often fail because the cement lute breaks down as a result of constant flexion between the implant and the

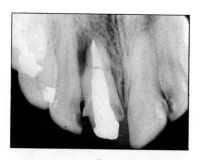

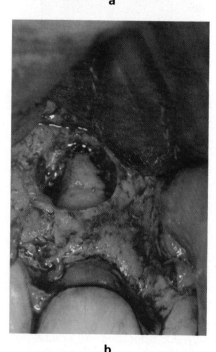

Figure 12.7 a, *Fracture 1 , as revealed on a bisecting angle radiograph.* **b,** *At operation the fracture shown in* **(a)** *was found to extend obliquely so far downwards and palatally that correction was impossible*

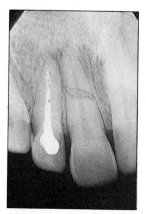

Figure 12.6 *An oblique fracture, as seen on a long-cone radiograph (simulated)*

periodontally weakened root. This problem can partly be overcome by the use of a strong, adhesive, insoluble cement, such as the epoxy-resin based AH-26; and by splinting the stabilized tooth to one of its more secure neighbours (Figures 12.8 and 12.9). An oblique fracture will expose the root canal in some part of its coronal length. At this level, the diameter of the canal will often be too great to allow instrumentation to a circular shape that will allow the precise fit of a matched endodontic implant (Figure 12.10). In such instances there is inevitably an excess of cement lute between the implant and

the canal wall, and the use of an insoluble material, such as AH-26, is again recommended. Attempts may also be made to plug the defect with silver amalgam.

The prognosis of a stabilized tooth is particularly poor if part of the fracture terminates close to the epithelial attachment at the base of the gingival crevice (Figures 12.11 and 12.12). Very little apical migration of the epithelial attachment need occur before there is a direct communication between the mouth and the implant, with consequent infection of the alveolar bone and inevitable loss of the tooth.

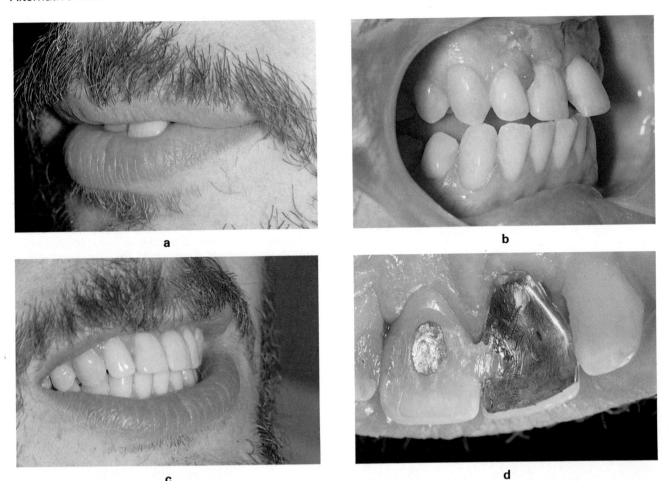

Figure 12.8 *Treatment of fractured 1| and non-vital, proclined, |1. **a, b,** |1 crown was fractured as the result of an accident, and was restored with a post crown by the general dental practitioner. Following restoration the tooth progressively proclined, worsening as the lip became trapped. **c,** A retrograde amalgam seal was placed above the post |1, and the tooth was retracted orthodontically. The fractured root apex 1| was removed and an endodontic splint placed, being cemented with AH-26. 1|1 were splinted. The case was stable after 4 years. **d,** Composite splint 1|1 (mirror image)*

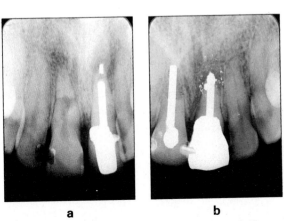

Figure 12.9 a, *Preoperative radiograph of the case illustrated in Figure 12.8.* **b,** *1 year postoperatively*

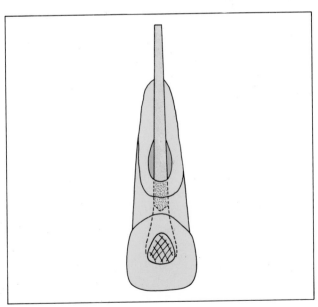

Figure 12.10 *It may not be possible to achieve an accurate fit of a matched stabilizer to the canal of an obliquely fractured root; consequently, excess cement lute will be exposed*

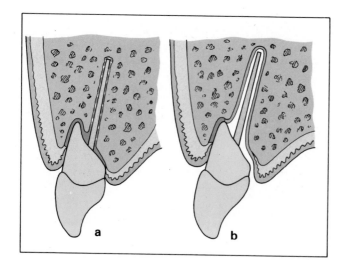

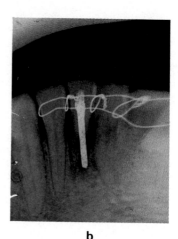

Figure 12.11 *The most coronal part of an obliquely fractured root may lie close to the epithelial attachment* **(a)**. *Little apical migration need occur before epithelium surrounds the implant and infection of the supporting tissues supervenes* **(b)**

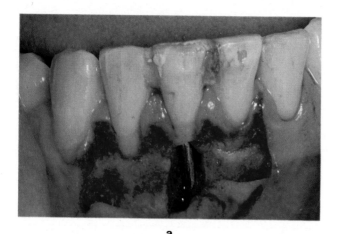

a

b

Figure 12.12 a, *Treatment of an oblique fracture. Endodontic implant placed in lower central incisor.* **b,** *Immediate postoperative radiograph. The implant is rather short. However, failure after 18 months was caused by infection resulting from the lack of an epithelial attachment to the very short length of remaining buccal root surface*

Chapter 13

Postoperative Appointment; Review and Assessment; Restoration

Following surgery, and as soon as postoperative symptoms have resolved, the access cavity must be permanently filled. Weakened cusps should be protected with semipermanent restorations, such as the useful intracoronal etched-enamel composite splint (Figure 13.1). The patient may be informed that it is usually possible to start definitive restorative treatment following the first review appointment in about 6 months. It is often sensible to take a realistic chance, and place a definitive restoration sooner, on the assumption that healing will proceed satisfactorily.

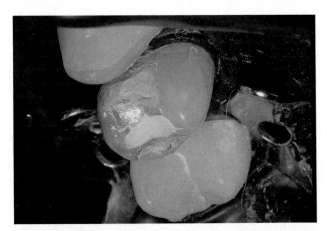 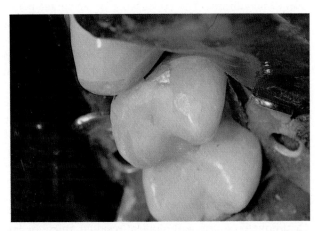

Figure 13.1 *Intracoronal composite splint. The internal enamel walls have been etched, but note that not all the original restoration needs to be removed*

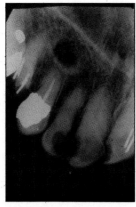

Figure 13.2 *Radiolucency caused by loss of cortical plate following an apicectomy. The periodontal membrane can be traced intact around the root end*

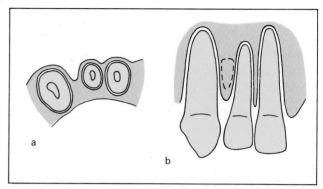

Figure 13.3 *A deep hollow between two roots can cause a radiolucency that mimics a lateral cyst*

Review and Assessment

The apicectomy should be reviewed about 6 months postoperatively, although the patient must be advised to seek advice in the interim, should signs or symptoms supervene.

Signs and symptoms

A history of severe symptoms, or the presence of signs, such as a sinus, deep periodontal pocketing, and/or undue mobility, indicate that the apicectomy has failed. In the absence of signs and symptoms, the assessment of success or failure must be made on the basis of radiographic evidence.

Radiographic assessment

Resolution of apical area

Apical bony defects, even when substantial, should be expected to repair within 6 months, certainly a year, at which time there should be radiographic evidence of the reformation of cancellous bone, lamina dura and periodontal membrane. The appearance of an intact periodontal membrane can, however, be misleading, and this will be discussed later. Treatment may usually be considered to have failed when an apical lesion either has not substantially reduced in size, or has increased in size.

It is unwise to make an irrevocable decision on the basis of a single follow-up radiograph, because of the variations in image density that can occur as a result of slight differences in exposure time and developing procedure.

Apical radiolucencies not requiring treatment

Occasionally, a non-pathological residual apical or lateral radiolucency may be misdiagnosed and interpreted

as a sign of failure, with the risk of further, unnecessary surgical intervention.

Loss of cortical plate as a result of previous surgery (Figure 13.2). This usually occurs as the result of heavy-handed dentistry, too much bone having been removed at the time of surgery. The periodontal membrane and lamina dura can usually be traced around the tip of the apicected tooth, the lesion being discretely sited in the adjacent bone. The appearance is particularly clearcut when a communication exists between the soft tissues on both sides of the alveolus.

Where the alveolar bone and cortical plate dip deeply to form a hollow between two prominent root eminences (Figure 13.3). The radiographic appearance is similar to that of a lateral cyst. The diagnosis is usually apparent as soon as the mucoperiosteal flap is raised, and further intervention is unnecessary.

Scar tissue. Apical lesions may occasionally be found, on histological examination, to consist of dense, fibrous scar tissue, associated with a small amount of chronic inflammatory cell infiltration. The absence of signs and symptoms, and often a history of repeated surgical intervention will suggest the diagnosis (Figure 13.4). No treatment is required.

Fibrous repair associated with an amalgam seal. Gutta-percha appears to be well tolerated by the tissues. Silver amalgam causes a mild inflammatory response (Figure 13.5), and consequently amalgam seals are usually isolated from the surrounding alveolar bone by a narrow 'capsule' of fibrous tissue. This capsule may be visible on a radiograph if the X-ray beam passes tangential to the surface of the seal, as, for example, in the case of a mesial or distal perforation repair (Figure 13.6). Evidence of fibrous repair is less often observed above apical amalgam seals because the lesion is obscured by superimposition of the more deeply placed, obliquely angled portion of the cut root-tip (Figure 13.7). It is

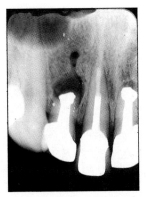

Figure 13.4 *Apicected 2| . Radiograph taken 2 years after the fifth (and last) intervention. The tooth was symptomless and there were no signs. There had been some resolution since the immediate postoperative radiograph was taken. The radiolucent area was diagnosed as scar/chronic infective tissue*

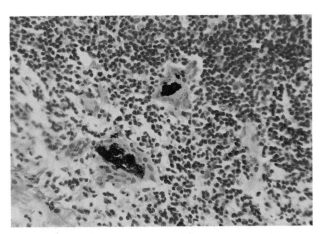

Figure 13.5 *Amalgam tattoo. The black silver (sulphide) particles are surrounded by fibrous and chronic inflammatory cells*

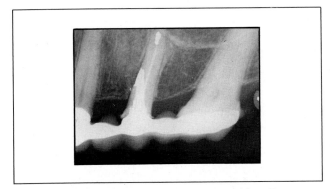

Figure 13.6 *Repair of mesial perforation. One year postoperatively. A narrow 'capsule' can be seen to lie between the amalgam seal and the bone*

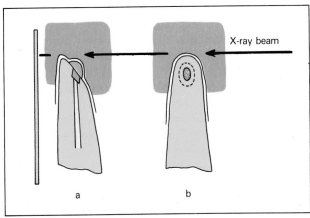

Figure 13.7 *Fibrous tissue lying above an apical seal is often obscured on radiographs by superimposition of the more deeply placed root. The periodontal membrane appears to run intact, around the root-tip*

usually the periodontal membrane and lamina dura lying above the most apical part of the cut root that are clearly defined on the X-ray, and which give the false impression of complete healing. The X-ray beam will sometimes pass tangentially to the cut surface of an apicected root (usually when a horizontal resection has been made). A small apical radiolucency will usually be observed in such cases (Figure 13.8), and should not be interpreted as a sign of failure, except in the presence of symptoms or signs.

There are many other causes of apically related radiolucencies. Some of these are pathological in nature. Others simply represent the superimposition or close relationship of a normal anatomical feature – for example, the incisive foramen (Figure 13.9), the mental foramen or the maxillary antrum. The subject is well covered in specialist radiographic and endodontic textbooks.

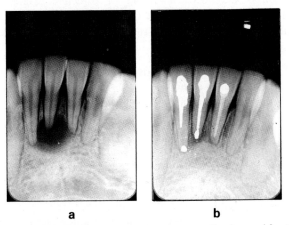

a   **b**

Figure 13.8 *Apicectomy; **a**, preoperatively and **b**, 10 months postoperatively. The small radiolucencies at the root-tips were considered, in the absence of signs and symptoms, to be scar tissue*

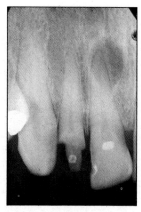

Figure 13.9 *Superimposition over the root apex, of the incisive canal (cystic?)*

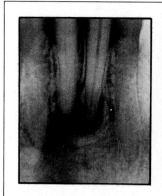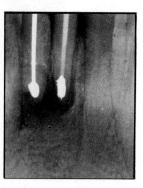

Figure 13.10 *Apicectomy; preoperatively and 2 years postoperatively. The radiolucent area was not associated with visible signs, but the patient complained of occasional discomfort. The radiolucency almost certainly indicates the presence of chronic infective tissue. It is difficult to see what further treatment might be undertaken.*

Unresolved apical lesions requiring further investigation

Large apical lesions that fail to resolve, or lesions that have increased in size, must be investigated, and the decision to intervene is clearcut. Smaller lesions can, however, pose a considerable diagnostic and management problem.

Some patients will complain of occasional pain from an apicected tooth, occurring particularly when their general health is at a low ebb. There are seldom visible signs, but radiographs will usually show evidence of incomplete healing at the root apex (Figure 13.10). Such lesions contain acute or chronic inflammatory cells and must be distinguished from the small fibrous scars that are usually associated with amalgam seals. Rud and Andreasen have suggested that whereas scars are limited to the cut apical tip (Figure 13.8 and Figure 13.11a), chronic infective lesions will be seen on radiographs to extend around the lateral walls of the root – a useful diagnostic criterion (Figure 13.10 and Figure 13.11b). Further surgical intervention may be required if the lesion is diagnosed as being of infective origin. If further treatment is deemed not to be possible, the tooth may be retained and kept under observation, provided that:

(1) the symptoms remain occasional and mild,
(2) there are no signs,
(3) the radiolucent area does not increase in size.

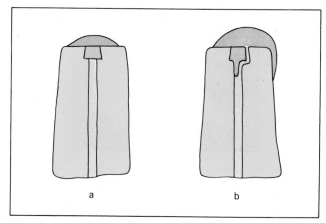

Figure 13.11 *Fibrous/scar tissue is usually limited to the area of the apical seal (a). Chronic infection tends to extend around the root-tip (b). See also Figure 13.10. (After Rud and Andreasen)*

Restoration of the Apicected Tooth

Posterior teeth

Apicectomy will usually have followed previous attempts at endodontic treatment, and frequently the crowns of teeth are weakened as the result either of large restorations or the preparation of access cavities. The remaining tooth structure should, whenever possible, be supported with a cast restoration that affords either cuspal or full coverage. Unfortunately, there is often so little remaining coronal tissue that a conservative restoration cannot be placed, and the weakened walls have to be sacrificed, function being restored by means of a crown supported on a post or pin retained core. Readers are referred to the appropriate texts. Prevention is, however, better than cure, and a light touch when cutting cavities, and a sparing removal of tissue when obtaining access, will greatly lessen future restorative problems.

Anterior teeth

Resection of too much root during apicectomy will reduce the length of root canal available for the retention of a post (Figure 13.12a). This problem can, to some extent, be overcome by reducing less of the crown during post and core preparation, so that additional

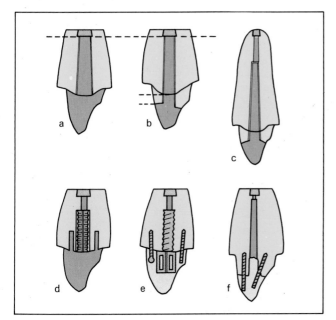

Figure 13.12 *Means of restoring a broken-down anterior tooth.* **a,** *Post and core. 'Rooftop' preparation.* **b,** *Post and core. Retention of sound coronal dentine.* **c,** *Post and core. Minimal root-tip has been resected and as much coronal dentine as possible retained.* **d,** *Cast grooved post, accessory pins and core.* **e,** *Preformed threaded post, accessory dentine pins and composite core.* **f,** *Dentine pins and composite core. Note that one-half the core length is comprised of substantial dentine*

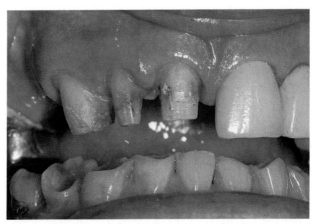

Figure 13.13 *Use of dentine pins to retain composite cores. Sufficient crown dentine remained for this technique to be successful. The teeth were vital. The lower arch was restored with an overlay denture*

retention is gained from the length of post situated within the remaining coronal tissue (Figure 13.12b). This advice ought to be unnecessary, in the light of current practice, for two reasons. First, a minimal length of root apex is normally resected, certainly never so much that the retention of a post is likely to be in jeopardy. Second, the reduction of residual crown tissue is always as conservative as possible. The old 'rooftop' preparation (Figure 13.12a) should never electively be cut, except in the absence of substantial coronal dentine. The ideal design for the post and core restoration of an apicected tooth is illustrated in Figure 13.12c.

Occasionally, the length of root canal available for post retention is unacceptably short; for example, as the result of an irremovable broken instrument or post. Such an obstruction can usually partly be burred out, but can seldom be cut away in sufficient length to allow preparation and cementation of a conventional cemented, tapered cast post. Increased retention can sometimes be gained in such cases by cementing a serrated, parallel-sided post. The Parapost System (Figure 13.12d) allows such a post to be cast in gold, together with additional parallel-sided wrought pins that serve both to 'splint' the root and gain additional retention. Alternatively, a preformed threaded post may be screwed and cemented into a tapped post hole. One such system is the Radix Anchor, which allows a composite core to be constructed, extra retention being gained, if necessary, from self-tapping dentine pins (Figure 13.12e).

If a post cannot be placed in the root canal, a pin-retained coping may be cast, or dentine pins alone can be used to provide retention for a composite core. Such a core will not, however, provide adequate support for an artificial crown in normal function, unless a substantial length of the overall crown preparation can be cut in sound tooth tissue (Figure 13.12f and Figure 13.13).

Reference

Rud, J. and Andreasen, J. O. (1972). *Endodontic Surgery.* (Copenhagen: Munksgaard)

Chapter 14

Correction of Failure (Re-apicectomy)

The criteria by which failure is judged were discussed in Chapter 13. The causes of failure fall into six principal groups, the boundaries of which are indistinct.

(1) Incompletely sealed root canals (the commonest cause of failure)

(2) Unidentified damage to the root (fracture, perforation)

(3) Deep periodontal pocketing

(4) Breakdown of the associated supporting tissues

(5) Adverse reaction to the apical sealant

(6) Inexplicable

Incompletely Sealed Root Canals

Unidentified root

An experienced operator should recognize the normal diameter of a single-rooted tooth resected at a given level. If the end of the cut root is atypically narrow, he should suspect that a second, more deeply placed root remains to be identified. Once the buccal root has been resected, the tip of a more deeply placed root will no longer be hidden as a result of superimposition, and it will be revealed on a radiograph exposed at the time of operation. Despite all precautions, additional roots are sometimes missed, and particularly in the case of upper first and second premolars should be considered as a likely cause of failure. Every effort should be made positively to identify suspected additional roots prior to re-apicectomy, by means of radiographs taken at different antero-posterior angles.

An unidentified root should be suspected as a cause of failure if, at re-entry, the apical seal in the resected root is found to be intact and the surrounding tissues well healed. Additional signs may be softening or breakdown of the interradicular bone as a result of infection arising from a deeply placed, undetected root.

Failure to completely resect and remove the root-tip

If the root-tip is incompletely resected and thus not removed, it is almost inevitable that some part of the root canal system will remain in direct communication with the supporting tissues and will be a likely cause of failure (*see* Figure 6.7b and c, page 38).

Failure to completely obturate the root canal

The placement of a simple retrograde seal, leaving the bulk of the root canal uncleansed and unfilled, is a common cause of apicectomy failure (Figure 14.1). Re-apicectomy will usually prove successful, provided that the root canal is cleansed and obturated.

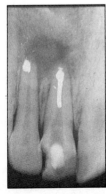

Figure 14.1 *Failure of retrograde apicectomy, caused almost certainly because the root canals had not properly been cleansed or obturated*

Imperfect apical seal

The apical seal may be found, at reoperation, to be imperfect.

There are five usual causes:

(1) An unidentified root canal (Figure 14.2)

(2) A circular filling point cemented into a non-circular canal with subsequent solution of the luting material (*see* Figure 1.5, page 11)

(3) An incompletely run-out apical cavity, in a narrow, irregular terminal root canal (Figure 14.3)

(4) An insufficiently condensed apical seal

(5) An apical seal contaminated by blood or saline

The usual reason for perpetrating the errors listed above is the failure properly to expose the root-tip at the time of operation, with the result that the root canals are not positively identified. Uncontrollable bleeding may also obscure vision and contaminate the field, and is another cause of failure. The necessary corrective measures are obvious.

Damage to the Root

Unidentified perforation (or large lateral canal)

The presence within a root canal of a post should always lead to the suspicion of an unidentified perforation. Bone loss usually occurs rapidly following perforation, and mesial or distal lesions can usually be diagnosed early by means of radiographs. Buccal and palatal bone loss can remain unidentified for a long time. Access to an area of palatal bone loss can sometimes be made by further resection of the root-tip, or by the removal of interstitial bone. Careful exploration with a Briault probe may allow the perforation or the extruded post to be identified. In many cases of palatal perforation, immediate repair is not possible and identification serves only to confirm the need for a replantation or extraction.

Vertical root fracture

Vertical root fractures are not often seen on radiographs, but must be suspected when a competently undertaken apicectomy fails for no apparent reason. Vertical fractures may occur as a result of stress applied by way of a post; following the overenthusiastic use of lateral spreaders during root filling; or, in posterior teeth, because the tooth crown is unduly weakened as a result of restoration (Figure 14.4). A careful examination should be made of the coronal margins of the root, particularly at the junction with a post and core (Figure 14.5), which will often have become loosened as a result of the fracture. Removal of the post and core will usually allow a diagnosis to be made.

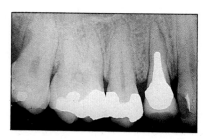

b

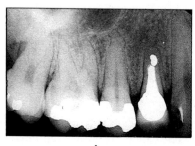

a

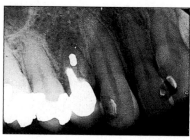

c

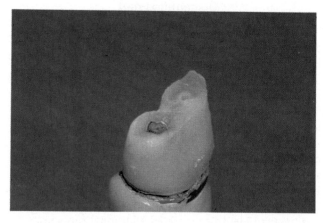

d

Figure 14.2 *Failed apicectomy 4|.* **a,** *Preoperatively.* **b,** *8 months postoperatively.* **c,** *1 year postoperatively (rotated view).* **d,** *Extracted tooth. Note that palatal canal remains unsealed. Had two differently angled preoperative radiographs been taken, or had* **c** *been properly studied, both roots could have been identified and filled, and extraction would probably not have been necessary. Reported case*

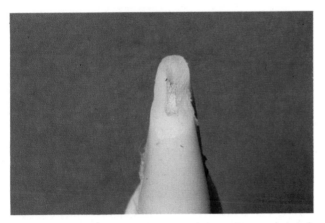

Figure 14.3 *A long narrow canal must be completely run-out and sealed (simulated)*

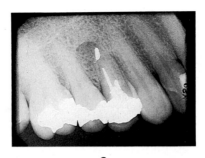

a

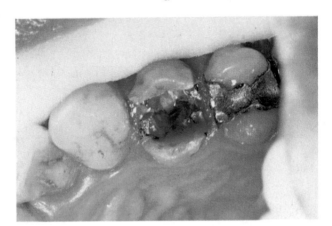

b

Figure 14.4 a, *Apicectomy* 4|, *6 months postoperatively. The radiolucency, for the treatment of which the operation was undertaken, remains.* **b,** *Removal of the amalgam filling revealed a vertical root fracture (mirror image)*

Cracks should also be sought, at the time of operation, in the apical length of root, where they present as a thin, darkly stained line, against which a sharp probe will usually catch. The diagnosis may be confirmed and the extent of the crack gauged by carefully removing a small amount of bone from the upper part of the root-face.

It is particularly difficult to identify a vertical fracture in the palatal aspect of the root. Provided that access is sufficient, careful searching with a sharp probe may detect a catch. It is usually necessary to make the diagnosis on the basis of deduction rather than observation.

In my opinion, vertical root fractures in the non-vital single-rooted tooth cannot be treated, other than by extraction.

Horizontal and oblique root fractures

Oblique root fractures can usually be identified by means of careful radiographic examination. Treatment is discussed in Chapter 12.

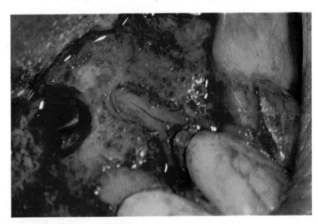

Figure 14.5 *Vertical root fracture* |3. *The post and core had been recemented several times*

Diagnostic signs

There are two signs which, when seen together, are diagnostic either of root perforation or root fracture: first, a sinus placed coronal and lateral to the underlying root apex (Figure 14.6); second, radiographic evidence of lateral bone loss. In the case of early perforations this bone loss is localized and circumscribed (Figure 14.7). Vertical root fractures usually cause the loss of bone along a greater length of root (Figure 14.8).

Deep Periodontal Pocketing

Resection of too great a length of root might, conceivably, in the presence of periodontal pocketing, result in the eventual loss of the tooth, as the consequence of insufficient periodontal support. More usually, it is the reduced distance between the epithelial attachment and the root end that constitutes the greatest risk of failure.

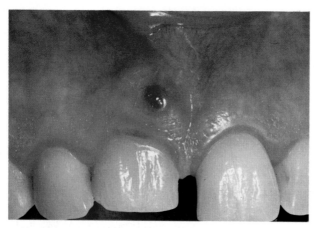

Figure 14.6 *Low level sinus, indicating an underlying root fracture; the result of trauma*

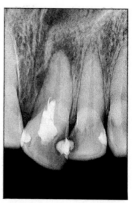

Figure 14.7 *Lateral radiolucency, typically indicating the presence of a recent root perforation*

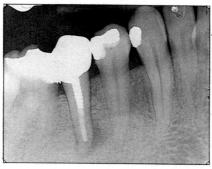

a

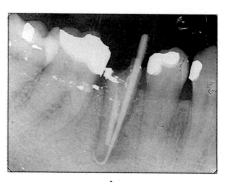

b

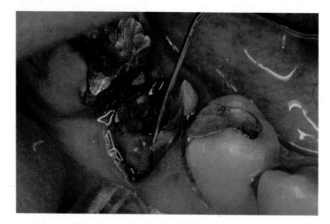

c

Figure 14.8 a, *Apical radiolucency associated with $\overline{5|}$. **b,** Subsequent investigation shows the presence of a lateral sinus and extensive longitudinal bone loss, diagnostic of a longitudinal fracture. **c,** Removal of the crown confirms the diagnosis of a root fracture. (Radiographs and transparencies reproduced by kind permission of Dr G. Lavagnoli, MD, FICD, Milan)*

Little further breakdown and migration of the epithelial attachment need occur in order to create a full length pocket extending from the mouth to the apical tissues (Figure 14.9).

A full length pocket can also develop as a consequence of drainage along the root-face of pus arising in the apical tissues (Figures 14.10a, b). Deep pocketing to the apex is sometimes difficult to diagnose, but must be considered as a cause of otherwise inexplicable apicectomy failure, infection of the apical tissues being maintained from the mouth by way of the pocket. The condition is discussed further in Chapter 16.

Breakdown of the Associated Supporting Tissues

The periodontal, alveolar and gingival tissues may break down as a consequence of unsuccessful apical surgery. Treatment of the condition is considered in Chapters 16 and 17.

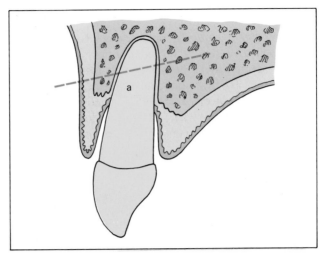

Figure 14.9 *Very little of the root-tip need be resected in the presence of deep pocketing, to allow a communication between the mouth and the apical tissues*

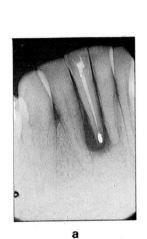

a

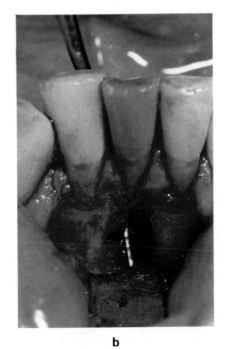

b

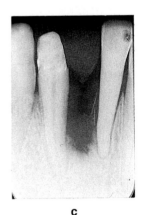

c

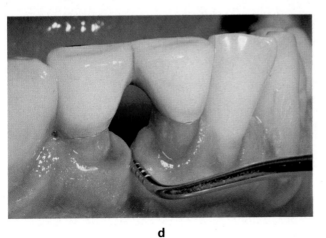

d

Figure 14.10 *Apicectomy 7|. Deep lingual pocketing caused by longstanding apical infection (a, b) could not be eliminated. c, Upon extraction the extent of the bone loss was found to be considerable. d, A two-unit 'bridge' was made to allow thorough cleansing of the gingival margins 2|1*

Adverse Reaction to the Apical Sealant

Silver amalgam causes a mild foreign body reaction when used as a sealant in endodontic surgical procedures. Attempts have been made to identify suitable sealants that are more bio-compatible. Cohesive gold, glass ionomer cements, zinc oxide/eugenol and composite resin have all been tried and (to date) found wanting. Currently amalgam remains the material of necessity, if not of choice. Despite its mild irritant effect, the use of amalgam is unlikely to cause an apicectomy to fail, provided that:

(1) the material is contained within the root canal,
(2) the surface area of the seal is kept as small as possible,
(3) the exposed surface of the amalgam is burnished in order to reduce the surface roughness (Figures 14.11 a–d),
(4) the amalgam is uncontaminated with saline or blood.

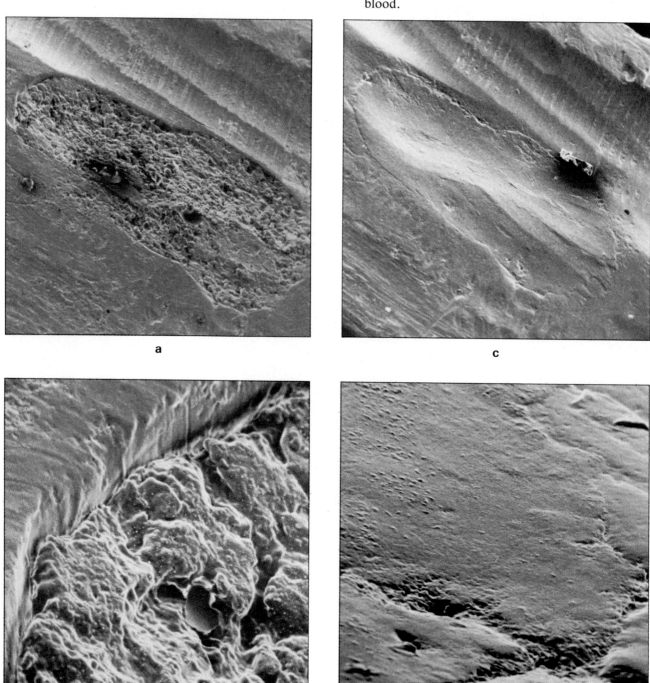

a

c

b

d

Figure 14.11 *Scanning electron micrographs of lathe-cut amalgam seal.* **a, b,** *Unburnished;* **c, d,** *Burnished with a ball-ended burnisher. Fields of view 3.5 mm; 350 μm. (Replicas photographed by courtesy of Professor A. Boyde, University College, London)*

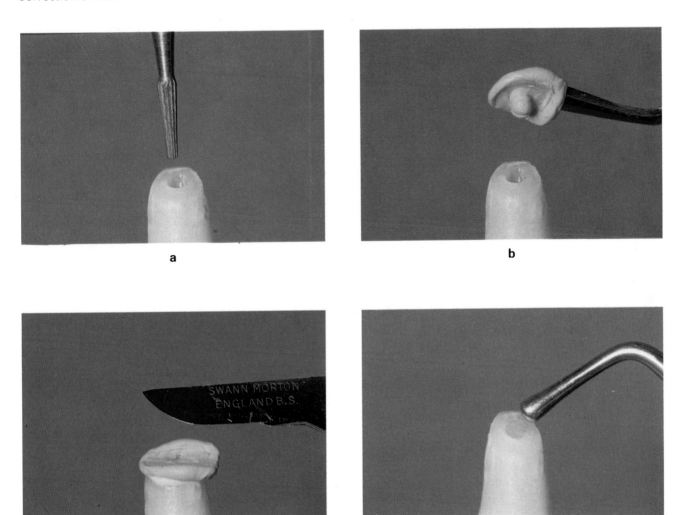

Figure 14.12 *Insertion of apical gutta-percha seal (after Andreasen).* **a,** *Preparation of cavity.* **b,** *Impression in warm gutta-percha.* **c,** *Cementation with Tubliseal of gutta-percha 'inlay', and reduction to the level of the root surface.* **d,** *Warm burnishing of gutta-percha seal*

The greater the length of root that is resected, the larger will be the area of amalgam in contact with the tissues. In extreme cases, such as that illustrated in Figure 13.4, page 91, it has proved beneficial to re-enter the site in order to polish the hardened surface of the abnormally large amalgam seal.

Andreasen suggested that an adverse reaction to amalgam should be considered as a cause of apicectomy failure, if no other reason can be found. He recommended that in such cases the amalgam seal be replaced by a gutta-percha inlay. The technique is illustrated in Figure 14.12 a–d. The development of the thermoplastic gutta-percha systems now affords another method of placing a gutta-percha retrograde seal. I have had little success using gutta-percha as a retrograde seal. However, the teeth on which the technique was used were being treated for a second or third time and it is

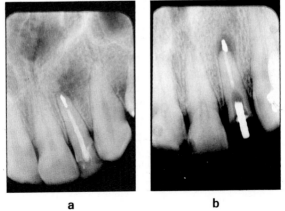

Figure 14.13 *Apicectomy* ⌊2. **a,** *Immediately postoperatively.* **b,** *1 year postoperatively. The root-tip has resorbed from around the amalgam seal*

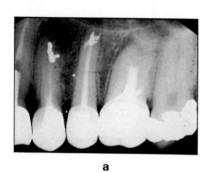 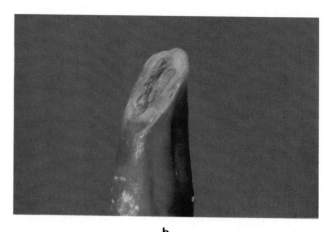

a · b

Figure 14.14 *Apicectomy* ⌊*45. The patient presented with a mouth of appalling root fillings. Despite two apparently adequate apicectomies* ⌊*45 had to be extracted because of continuous apical infection. Upon extraction, the root was seen tobe highly stained* **(b)**, *suggesting deep contamination of the dentinal tubules, possibly by a formalin-containing root canal sealant*

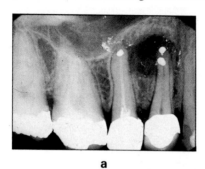 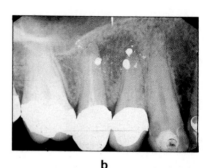

a · b

Figure 14.15 a, b, *Apicectomy* 54⌋ *. Immediately postoperatively, and 1 year postoperatively. Apical seal* 5⌋ *has 'migrated'. An insufficient undercut in the apical cavity is a rare cause of apicectomy failure*

possible that they were unsaveable by any means, perhaps as a consequence of deep bacterial or chemical contamination of the dentine surface.

Inexplicable

An apicectomy may sometimes fail for no apparent reason (Figure 14.13). Causes can be postulated, for example deeply penetrative or abnormally pathogenic bacterial or chemical contamination of the root dentine (Figure 14.14). Often all that can be done is to re-apicect, in the hope that the cause of failure will be eliminated.

When an apicectomy has failed, a decision must be made as to whether the patient should be subjected to more surgery. Much will depend upon the need to retain the tooth and, importantly, upon the wishes of the patient.

We all make mistakes (Figure 14.15), and it is reasonable to hope that a second attempt will throw light upon an earlier error. However, if an experienced operator is certain that every care has been taken in his first two attempts, it is difficult to see what advantage is to be gained from a third. Referred patients, some of whom may have suffered three or more unsuccessful interventions, pose a particular problem. The decision to intervene yet again must be made on the basis of a thorough clinical examination, and the exercise of commonsense, and occasionally tact.

Reference

Andreasen, J. O. (1982). Communication, Joint meeting, British Endodontic Society/British Paedodontic Society

Chapter 15

Equipment

Most practitioners will have an established preference for particular surgical instruments. The surgical set-up illustrated in Figure 15.1 is the one that I use and is shown simply as a guide. The bulb syringe is now no longer used and has been replaced with a disposable plastic syringe.

Sterility

Apicectomy wounds rarely become seriously infected. This good fortune should not be considered a reason for not using a sterile technique.

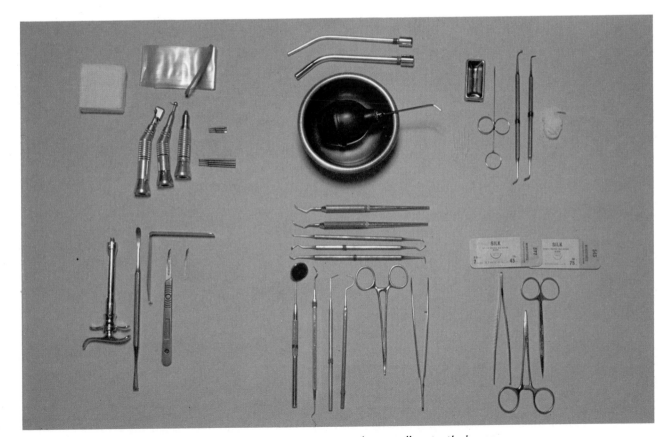

Figure 15.1 *Surgical set-up. The instruments are grouped according to their use*

All surgical equipment can nowadays be sterilized – including handpieces and some motors, which can be autoclaved. Those motors and cables that cannot be autoclaved should be sheathed at the time of operation, in a length of sterile plastic tubing (Figure 15.2). The ends of tubing can be kept patent during autoclaving by the insertion of two lengths of ribbon gauze, which may themselves be used during the operation. Surgical gloves must be worn.

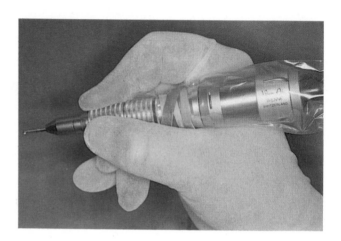

Figure 15.2 *Handpiece and electromotor. The unsterilizable electromotor and cable are sleeved at the time of operation with a length (ca. 70 cm) of thin autoclaved plastic tubing. (Lay Flat Nylon Film, 810/030/050, Portex Ltd, available from Southern Syringes Ltd, Unit L3, Lyntown Trading Estate, Lynwell Road, Eccles, Manchester M30 9GN)*

Chapter 16

Periodontal Considerations I

Damage to the periodontal and supporting tissues may be seen in association with a non-vital tooth that is to be, or which has been, apicected. Damage may occur preoperatively as a consequence of the apical lesion that is to be treated (Figure 16.1a). Alternatively, the breakdown may be iatrogenic: the result of unsuccessful surgery (Figure 16.1b)

The Supporting Tissues in Health

A brief account of the periodontal supporting tissues is given in order to clarify the later texts (Figure 16.2).

At the base of the gingival crevice the innermost cells of the junctional epithelium are attached by means of hemidesmosomes, either to the most apical part of the enamel surface, or usually in the adult tooth to cementum at the coronal part of the root (Figure 16.3) Apical to the gingival attachment, bundles of collagen fibres pass from the periodontal membrane into the cementum, where they spread laterally beneath the surface. The collagen fibres form a major part of the periodontal membrane and are attached laterally to the bone of the socket, the crestal bone and the gingival submucosa.

Periodontal Disease

The formation of a periodontal pocket is associated with apical migration of the epithelial attachment, breakdown of the periodontal fibre attachment and a concomitant resorption of alveolar bone. A pocket thus comprises epithelium on its outer aspect, cementum on the inner (Figure 16.2b). The cementum is contaminated with bacteria and products of their metabolism, both of which play a major role in preventing the reattachment of fibroblasts or epithelial cells to the root surface.

Periodontal pocketing is treated by eliminating (as far as possible) extrinsic factors such as plaque. Intrinsic factors, for example, an exaggerated immune defence

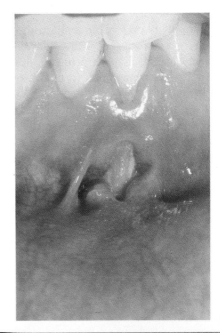

a

b

Figure 16.1 a, *Breakdown of the gingival tissues as a result of acute apical infection.* **b,** *Breakdown of the gingival tissues following unsuccessful apical surgery*

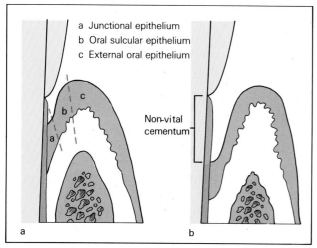

Figure 16.2 a, *Diagrammatic representation of the gingival attachment in health.* **b,** *Early periodontal pocketing. There has been ulceration, breakdown and apical migration of the epithelial attachment*

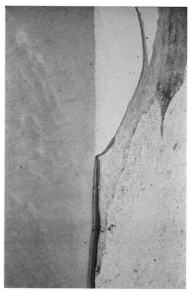

Figure 16.3 *Attachment of epithelium to the darkly staining cementum (centre field). The decalcified root dentine is on the left*

response, cannot at present be dealt with. Thorough debridement of the root-face will often allow the re-establishment of a soft tissue attachment, usually a long junctional epithelial attachment, formed as the result of a rapid downgrowth of cells (Figure 16.4b). It is probably the speed with which the epithelial cells migrate along the root-face that prevents the attachment of more slowly organizing fibroblasts.

A long junctional epithelial attachment is clinically acceptable in patients with satisfactory standards of plaque control, but nevertheless offers less support than a fibrous attachment. It is also particularly susceptible to breakdown in the presence of inflammation. Much

research has been done on means of delaying epithelial downgrowth in order to promote fibrous attachment. One of the most intensively studied techniques has been the application to the root-face of citric acid, which may be effective in three ways: (1) by detoxifying bacterial remnants, (2) by superficially decalcifying the root surface, thus exposing a fibre-rich layer that may promote the organization and attachment of fibroblasts and (3) by exposing and widening the dentinal tubules to form an open meshwork that is unfavourable to the downward growth of epithelium, and which may thus afford sufficient time to allow the organization and

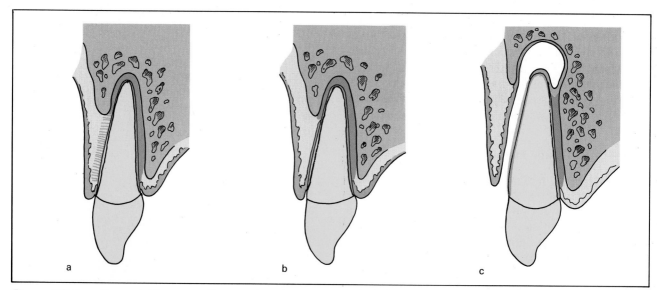

Figure 16.4 a, *Bony dehiscence. Connective tissue attachment between cementum and the overlying buccal gingival tissues.* **b,** *Bony dehiscence. The connective tissue attachment has been damaged following flap reflection. Attachment is now by means of a long epithelial junction.* **c,** *Contamination of the cementum prevents the reformation of an attachment, and an epithelialized pocket may be formed, extending from the gingival crevice to the root apex*

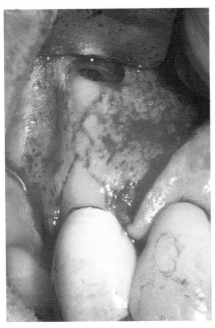

Figure 16.5 *Dehiscence 3| exposed during apicectomy. There was no previous pocketing, or evident contamination of the root cementum. The root is prominent and the adjacent bone thin. The dehiscence is probably naturally occurring*

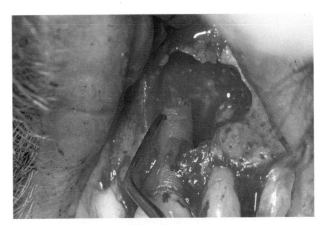

Figure 16.6 *Bony dehiscence arising as the result of longstanding apical infection*

attachment of fibrous cells. The results have been disappointing. Currently, efforts are being made to prevent epithelial downgrowth by the interpositioning on the root-face of membranes such as PTFE (Gore-Tex®). This means of achieving guided tissue regeneration shows promise, and worldwide clinical trials are currently being carried out.

Loss of the supporting tissues as a result of periodontal disease is not strictly comparable to the loss of such tissues as the result of apical infection and, although the factors that have been discussed offer guidance, they must be extrapolated with extreme caution.

Damage to the Periodontal Supporting Tissues as a Result of Apical Infection or Apical Surgery

Four conditions may occur.

(1) Bony dehiscences and fenestrations, not associated with infection and unrelated to mucosal breakdown. Such lesions are not manifestations of damage but are conveniently discussed at this stage

(2) Bony fenestrations and dehiscences arising as a result of infection but not associated with mucosal breakdown

(3) Localized breakdown of apically related mucosa and associated supporting tissues, as a result of infection

(4) Extensive breakdown of mucosa and associated supporting tissues as a result of infection. Gingival clefting

'Naturally occurring' bony fenestrations and dehiscences

Bony fenestrations or dehiscences are often found over the roots of healthy teeth (Figure 16.5), particularly lower lateral incisors and the mesio-buccal root of upper first molars. The defect may be the consequence of a disproportionately wide, or buccally inclined root. If the buccal plate is particularly thin, the inevitable bone loss that follows the raising of a muco-periosteal flap may lead to the subsequent formation of a bony dehiscence beneath the healed mucosa. The periodontal support is not unduly weakened by such dehiscences.

The nature of the periodontal attachment to that part of the root surface exposed by a dehiscence is poorly described. It may be assumed that collagen fibres pass from the cementum to intermingle with similar fibres lying in the overlying corium or submucosa (Figure 16.4a). These attachment fibres will be torn when a flap is raised but, provided that they are not further traumatized during surgery, will probably repair to reform a fibrous connective tissue attachment, following replacement and healing of the flap. The exposed root surface is not contaminated and *should not therefore be planed,* in a misguided attempt at debridement. If this is done, the torn fibres will be removed from the root face, and the flap will probably heal with the formation of a (less desirable) long epithelial attachment (Figure 16.4b).

Factors that indicate a dehiscence to be 'naturally occurring' are the prominence of the root, the thinness of the adjacent alveolar bone, and the absence of signs denoting infection (*see* below).

Bony fenestrations and dehiscences caused by infection

Pus formed in the apical tissues will usually break through the alveolar bone and mucosa, to form a buccal or lingual/palatal sinus. Occasionally, however, pus

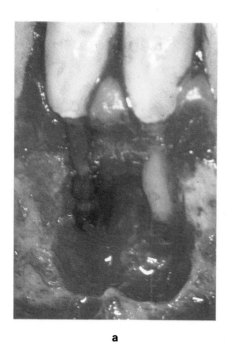

a

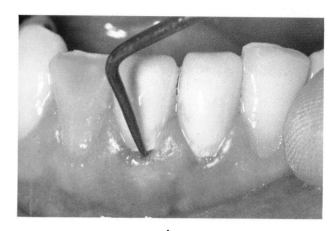

b

Figure 16.7 a, *Bony dehiscence* $\overline{1\,|1}$*. The root surface of* $\overline{1|}$ *is grossly contaminated and was thoroughly planed prior to closure of the flap.* **b,***One year postoperatively, following thorough mechanical planing of root surface* $\overline{1|}$ *. There were no signs or symptoms. Radiologically healing was satisfactory. Pocketing could not be identified*

tracks down the periodontal membrane. Such drainage will, if chronic, result in destruction of the periodontal membrane and the adjacent alveolar bone, with the consequent formation of a deep epithelium-lined pocket that extends from the gingival margin to the infected apical tissues. If the overlying alveolar plate is thin, or if the drainage is of long standing, a bony dehiscence may form (Figures 16.4c, 16.6 and 16.7). Such dehiscences can usually be distinguished from naturally occurring dehiscences by one or more of the following criteria:

(1) the presence of deep periodontal pocketing, identifiable by careful preoperative probing with a fine diagnostic instrument,

(2) staining of the cementum, or the accretion on its surface of dark seruminal-type subgingival calculus (Figure 16.7a),

(3) divergence of the dehiscence as it extends apically to merge with an area of apical bone loss (Figures 16.6 and 16.7a),

(4) undermining of the alveolar bone at the margins of the dehiscence.

It is essential that a pathologically created dehiscence is identified as such, and that the contaminated cementum and dentine is removed prior to closure of the flap (Figures 16.6 and 16.7). Reattachment is unlikely to occur if this is not done, and the pocket will remain to constitute a probable cause of future failure, infection of the apical tissues being maintained from the mouth (*see* Figure 14.10, page 99).

The nature of the new attachment, formed following debridement and closure, is uncertain. It is feasible that in the case of a *narrow dehiscence* a fibrous attachment could re-establish, from the lateral aspects of the bony defect; a long epithelial attachment is, otherwise, more likely.

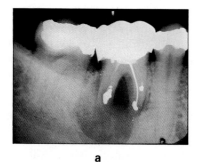

a

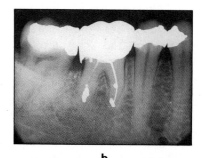

b

Figures 16.8 a, b, *Resolution of large apical area after 2 years, following the incomplete debridement of root surfaces and imperfect removal of pathological soft tissue. The apical seals were, however, sound*

Discussion

There is one condition where a fibrous attachment is probably re-established following the loss of supporting tissues, despite apparently ineffective debridement of the contaminated root-face, namely the large apical lesion. Longstanding apical infection can result in extensive destruction of apical supporting tissues. In many such cases the pus drains by way of a mucosal sinus and the epithelial attachment remains intact with an absence of pocketing. At operation, large areas of root surface are found to be denuded of bone, being covered with granulation tissue. It is seldom possible to achieve sufficient access to allow complete debridement of the root surfaces. Despite this, reformation of bone and re-establishment of a support mechanism will usually occur, provided that the root canals have been satisfac-

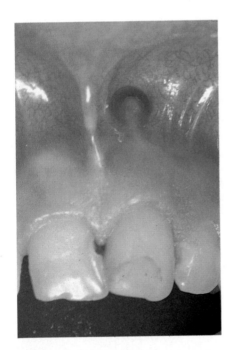

Figure 16.9 *Spontaneous resolution of an apical lesion following conventional root canal therapy. Case of Mr C. Hogg. (Reprinted by courtesy of the Editor of* Dental Update*)*

torily sealed (Figure 16.8). Perhaps in such circumstances the root surface is protected from bacterial contamination by an epithelial covering. Such a mechanism might account for the interesting case of a naturally healed apical lesion published in *Dental Update* by Mr C. Hogg (Figure 16.9).

The situation discussed above serves to illustrate fundamental differences between the loss of supporting tissue as a result of apical infection on the one hand, and periodontal disease on the other. The integrity of the epithelial attachment, the nature of the bacterial contaminants, variations in the tissue responses, are probably all important factors and require further investigation.

Limited breakdown of apical mucosa and associated supporting tissue

Mucosal breakdown and the exposure of a root-tip is a relatively infrequent complication of apical infection, but may occur if the root is buccally inclined (*see* Figures 16.1a and 16.10a). Resection of the exposed, contaminated root-tip may be all the treatment that is required, provided that a sufficient length of intact mucosa and sound periodontal support remains coronal to the fenestration. It is sensible to raise a full thickness envelope flap when treating such cases because it may be necessary to debride a length of the underlying root. A soft tissue deficiency will remain in the area of the fenestration following removal of the root-tip, and it is sensible to observe the natural healing over a period of a month or so, rather than immediately to attempt a complicated soft tissue repair (*see* Figures 16.10e and f).

Extensive breakdown of mucosa and underlying tissues

Extensive breakdown of the mucous membrane and underlying supporting tissues may occur buccally, in the anterior part of the lower jaw, as a consequence of three principal factors: (1) the thinness (or absence) of the alveolar bone overlying the upper part of the tooth roots, (2) the thinness and friability of the attached gingivae in this region and (3) the strong displacing force exerted on the mucosa by the deep fibres of the mentalis muscle (Figure 16.11). Although these factors increase the likelihood of breakdown, the initiating causes are usually acute apical infection (Figure 16.1a), or the unwise reflection of a mid-level flap (Figure 16.1b). In most instances the tissue loss is too extensive to allow treatment simply by resecting the exposed apical length of root, and complex periodontal repair procedures are required.

Gingival clefts may occur in either upper or lower jaw, and often arise as a result of vertical relieving incisions cut along the eminence of prominent roots (Figure 16.12).

Periodontal repair techniques are described in the following chapter.

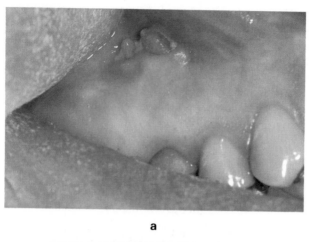

a

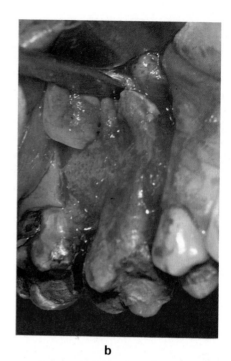

b

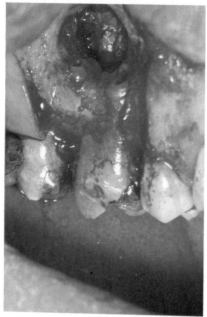

c

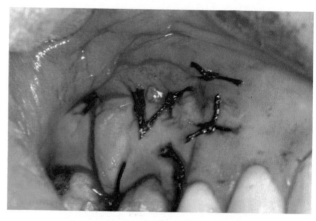

d

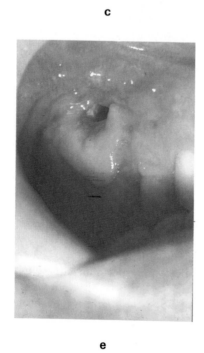

e

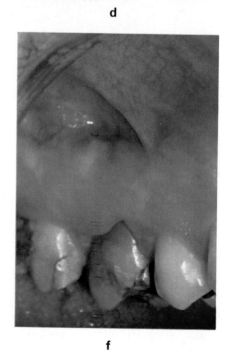

f

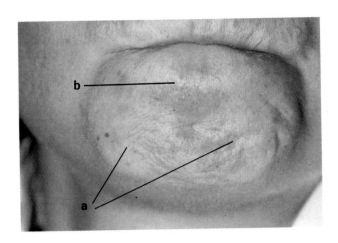

Figure 16.11 *The superficial fibres of the mentalis muscles are attached to the skin of the chin, and pucker the surface (a). The deep intercussating fibres press against and raise an underlying fibrous pad (b), placing strain upon overlying friable mucosal tissues*

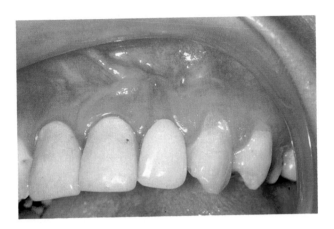

Figure 16.12 *Gingival cleft arising as a result of a vertical relief incision made at the crest of the gingival margin*

Figure 16.10 *Treatment of the buccal root-tips 6| , exposed as a result of acute apical infection. **a**, Preoperative appearance. **b**, Note the buccal inclination of the root-tips. **c**, Resection of root-tips and placement of apical seal (the palatal root was filled conventionally). **d**, Reapproximation of flap and repair of the mucosal perforation. **e**, Breakdown of repair after 1 week. **f**, Resolution of the mucosal breakdown as a result simply of irrigation and natural healing over a period of 4 months. (Case reproduced by courtesy of the Editor, International Endodontic Journal, and Mr W. L. Dawes)*

Chapter 17

Periodontal Considerations II

Mucosal breakdown
R. M. Palmer

Extensive mucosal breakdown may occur, particularly in the anterior part of the lower jar, prior to or as a result of apicectomy. In such cases, established periodontal techniques can be used to effect a repair. Two such cases are described.

Case 1

History

A 32-year-old woman presented with a gingival cleft extending to the apex $\overline{1|}$ (Figure 17.1). Apical surgery had previously been undertaken on $\overline{1|1}$, following which the wound had broken down, leaving the root exposed to the mouth for about 8 months. The apical seal $\overline{1|}$ was imperfect, and that in $\overline{|1}$ had been replaced to a satisfactory standard more recently, whilst the root-apex was exposed to the mouth.

Technique

A surgical technique was required to re-establish an apical seal in $\overline{1|}$, and to achieve soft tissue coverage of the denuded $\overline{|1}$ root. A laterally repositioned flap was used to correct this cleft. Care must be taken in designing such a flap so that its reapproximated sutured margins lie on sound, underlying bone. This is of particular importance where there are areas of apical bone loss associated with the deficiency that is to be repaired, as in the present case. An outline of the incisions is shown in Figure 17.2. They were comprised of an envelope flap raised from the gingival margin at $\overline{21|}$, in order to gain access to the apex $\overline{1|}$ (a, Figure 17.2); a pedicle flap (c, Figure 17.2), to be laterally positioned, outlined over $\overline{|23}$ (the donor site), and a 'U' shaped incision (b, Figure 17.2) placed between the two flaps and thus allowing the inflamed margins of the cleft to be excised.

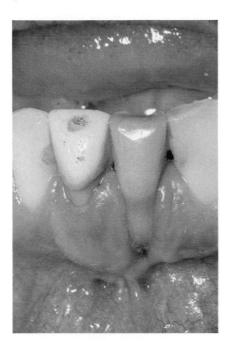

Figure 17.1 *Case 1 at presentation*

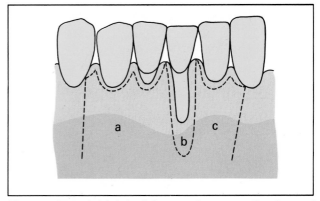

Figure 17.2 *Initial incisions prior to reflection of envelope flap (a) and pedicle flap (c). The margins of the cleft (b) were excised. The gingival incison is shown within the crevice*

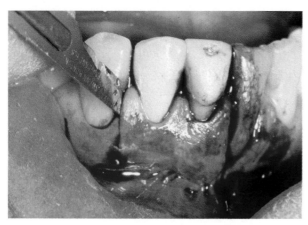

Figure 17.3 *Outline of envelope flap* $\overline{2\,1}$

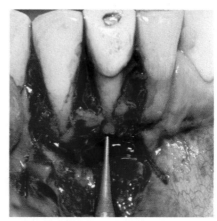

Figure 17.4 *Preparation of apical cavity* $\overline{1}$ *, to receive amalgam seal*

Procedure

Envelope flap $\overline{2\,1}$

The envelope flap (**a**, Figure 17.2), used to gain access for the apicectomy $\overline{1}$, was raised first, and is shown in Figure 17.3. The apex of $\overline{1}$ was prepared (Figure 17.4) and a new retrograde amalgam seal placed.

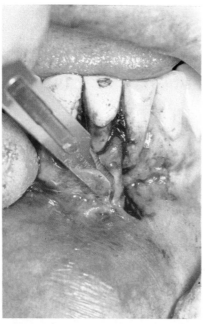

Figure 17.5 *Excision of right hand margin of cleft. Note the external bevel*

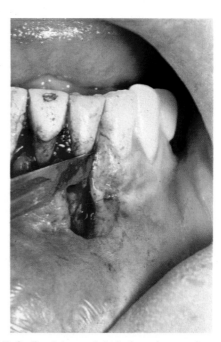

Figure 17.6 *Excision of left hand margin of cleft, with an internal bevel*

Excision of cleft margin. The margin of the gingival cleft was resected in order to provide fresh wound edges. The resection was extended sufficiently apically to remove the scar tissue that had formed as a result of previous surgery, in this way facilitating rotation of the pedicle flap. In excising the margins of the cleft, attempts were made to place an external bevel along the mesial incision of the envelope flap (Figure 17.5), and an internal bevel along the mesial incision of the pedicle flap (Figure 17.6), so that a halving joint was created on approximation of the two edges, following lateral replacement of the pedicle flap to its new site; thus facilitating healing.

The lateral flap $\overline{\smash{|3}}$

The laterally positioned pedicle flap was next raised, being extended to the mesial of $\overline{\smash{|3}}$ and including the entire papilla (Figure 17.7). It was thus wide enough to easily cover the defect. The incision at the gingival margin was made within the crevice (some operators prefer to employ an inverse bevel incision 1–2 mm from the gingival margin, thereby retaining a narrow cuff of tissue). The resected cleft and outline of the lateral flap are shown in Figure 17.8. The gingival part of the lateral flap was carefully raised in full thickness from the underlying alveolar bone, using a periosteal elevator, the mucosal element in part thickness by sharp dissection (Figure 17.9).

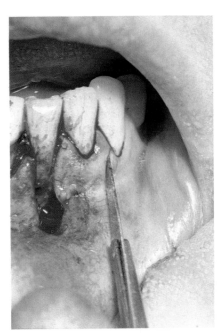

Figure 17.7 *The distal incision of the pedicle flap is made so as to include the whole interdental papilla* $\overline{\smash{|3}}$

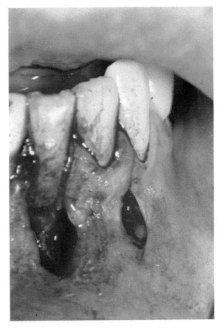

Figure 17.8 *Outline of the pedicle flap*

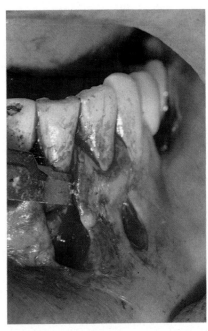

Figure 17.9 *Mucosal element of the pedicle flap is released by sharp dissection*

Elimination of the cleft

The exposed root surface that was to be covered by the graft was meticulously root-planed using sharp curettes (Figure 17.10). Figure 17.11 shows the released flaps in their natural position. In Figure 17.12 the lateral flap has been repositioned over the ⎯1⎯. It should be noted that the flap rests readily in its new position without tension. The flaps were sutured with 4/0 black silk, placed at the interdental papillae and along the vertical joint (Figure 17.13). Pressure was subsequently applied with damp gauze to maintain close adaptation and to stop bleeding. A periodontal pack was placed, which was removed at 10 days, as were the sutures (Figure 17.14).

The donor site, at which alveolar bone is exposed, heals by granulation and epithelialization, with minimal recession. In the early stages of healing, the patient should keep the surgical areas clean by gentle brushing and the use of Corsodyl mouthwash.

Review

The healed site at 3 months postoperatively is shown in Figure 17.15.

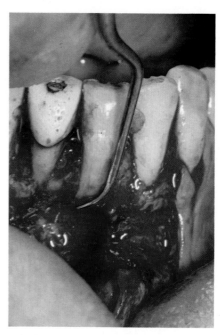

Figure 17.10 *Curettage of the denuded root-face*

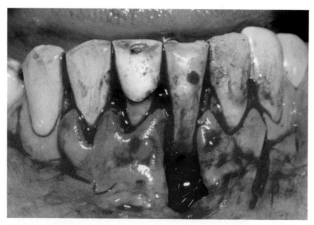

Figure 17.11 *Envelope and pedicle flap prior to replacement. Note the excision of the cleft margin*

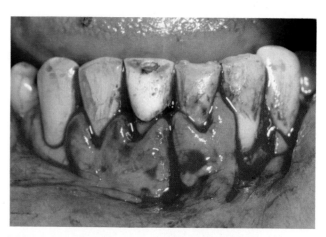

Figure 17.12 *Laterally positioned pedicle flap. The flap rests in its new site, without tension*

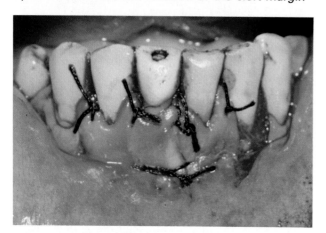

Figure 17.13 *Closure*

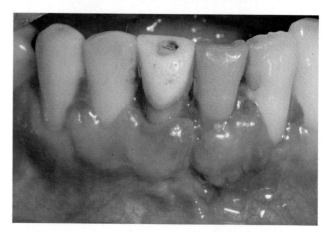

Figure 17.14 *Ten days postoperatively*

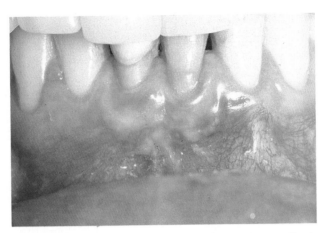

Figure 17.15 *Review. Three months postoperatively*

Case 2

History

The patient, a 23-year-old woman, presented with a mucosal defect overlying the apex of $\overline{1}$ (Figure 17.16), the consequence of an untreated apical abscess and a buccally inclined root-tip (Figure 17.17). A narrow band of marginal gingiva remained intact coronally, but was detached from the root surface, in effect forming an epithelialized bridge. $\overline{1}$ was also non-vital and radiographs showed there to be considerable bone loss around the apices of both teeth.

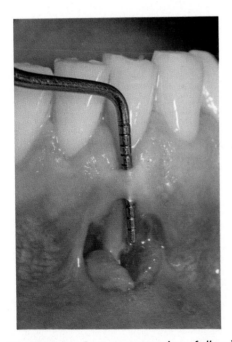

Figure 17.16 *Case 2 at presentation, following apical abscess 1 year previously. The base of the lesion comprised hyperplastic granulations. Coronally an epithelialized bridge spanned the cleft, but was unattached to the underlying root surface*

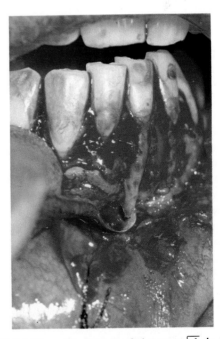

Figure 17.17 *The apical part of the root $\overline{1}$ is bucally inclined*

Technique

The deficiency was treated in the same way as the first case, described above. The margins of the cleft were excised, together with the detached gingival band and the large area of hyperplastic tissue at the base of the defect. An envelope flap was raised above $\overline{21}$ to allow a retrograde amalgam seal to be placed in $\overline{1|}$. A pedicle flap was raised at $\overline{|23}$. The contaminated, buccally inclined root $\overline{1|}$ was planed with slow speed burs, both to remove the contaminated surface layer and to produce a less prominent contour more conducive to mucosal healing (Figures 17.17 and 17.18). Following placement of an apical seal $\overline{|1}$, the pedicle flap was repositioned mesially, and sutured (Figure 17.19).

The 3-month postoperative appearance is shown in Figure 17.20. Some recession has occurred but the position is now stable.

Discussion

A laterally positioned flap is a pedicle graft which has a maintained blood supply and is, therefore, most suitable for placing on an avascular recipient site, such as a root surface. The most important prerequisite for such a procedure is a suitable donor site which, ideally, should comprise healthy gingival tissue of sufficient thickness, and with sound underlying bone. If there is insufficient alveolar bone at the donor site, recession may simply be transferred from recipient to donor site, although in some cases a therapeutic compromise may be justified.

The presence of prominent teeth and thin gingiva may suggest the presence of an underlying dehiscence at the donor site. Radiographs are of little help in determining the presence of a dehiscence, but careful exploratory probing under local anaesthesia can be diagnostic. Should a suitable donor site not be immediately available, one can be created by placing a free gingival graft apical to the defect. After a healing period of some months, the grafted tissue is positioned coronally to repair the defect.

Root surfaces exposed to prolonged plaque accumulation following an endodontically induced lesion, and those exposed as a result of chronic marginal periodontitis, are similar, in that both have lost their connective tissue attachment to the overlying tissues, and both have undergone surface alteration as a result of bacterial contamination. Meticulous root planing is essential if the root surface is to be rendered biologically acceptable to a graft.

From our present understanding of wound healing following periodontal surgery in the treatment of chronic inflammatory periodontal disease, it would seem that the most likely means of gaining attachment of the flap to the root surface is by way of a long junctional epithelium. The formation of a new connective tissue attachment of collagen fibres into cementum

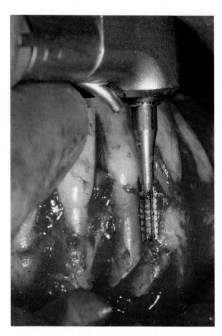

Figure 17.18 *Debridement and recontouring of the contaminated root-face*

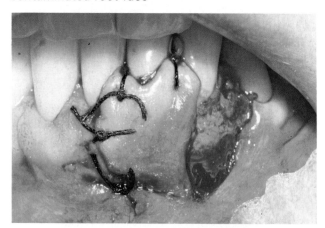

Figure 17.19 *Laterally repositioned flap. Note the donor site. Reflection of the coronally situated full thickness flap has exposed alveolar bone. Apically a part-thickness flap has been raised by sharp dissection*

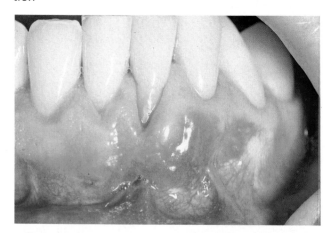

Figure 17.20 *Review. Three months postoperatively. Some recession has occurred but the condition is stable*

on the root surface is unlikely to be achieved. Studies in which citric acid has been used to demineralize the dentine surface in order to promote new attachment have not been universally successful and have in some cases resulted in resorption of the root surface. The use of surface conditioning agents is not recommended at the present time. From the clinical viewpoint a long junctional epithelium appears to be entirely satisfactory in the presence of good plaque control.

Treatment of amalgam tattoos
Principal author: D. G. Smith

Unsightly tattoos of the mucogingival tissues can arise as a consequence of the dispersal of silver amalgam within alveolar bone and soft tissues (Figure 17.21a). This complication is most likely to occur because amalgam has been retained within the bony cavity as a result of a poor sealing technique or as a result of inadequate debridement; or more frequently perhaps, as a result of the retention of fragments of amalgam beneath the apical parts of the flap, again the result of incomplete wound toilet. Should the condition be so extreme as to cause distress it can be treated by excising the unsightly discoloured tissues and repairing the defect by means of mucogingival surgery, such as the placement of a free mucosal graft. The technique is described below.

When amalgam tattoos encroach upon the gingival margin, alternative mucogingival procedures, such as pedicle flaps, may be necessary using techniques similar to those described earlier in this chapter for the repair of clefts.

Surgical technique

An illustrative case is shown in Figures 17.21 a–l and the surgical technique is described below.

Preparation of the recipient site

Following the administration of local anaesthetic solution, a template is prepared by trimming a piece of

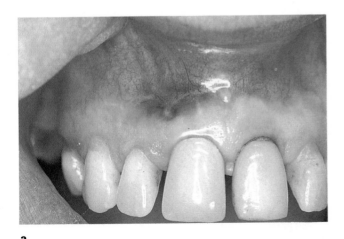

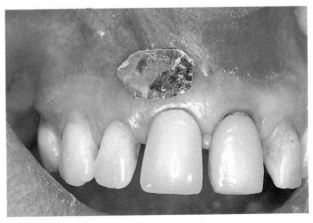

a

b

Figure 17.21 *continued overleaf*

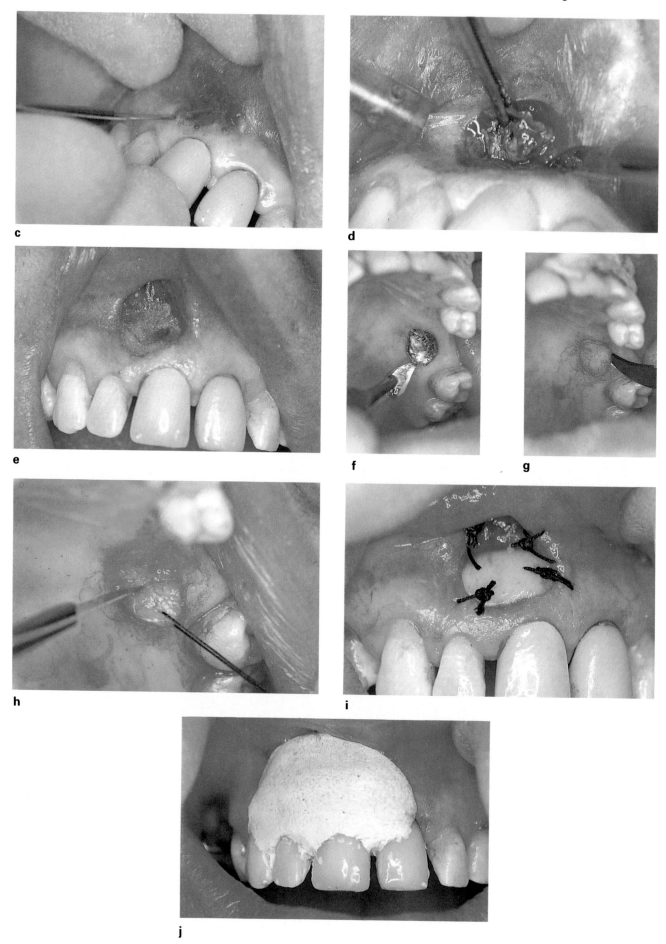

c

d

e

f

g

h

i

j

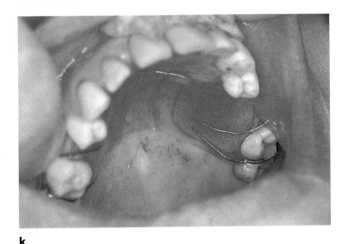

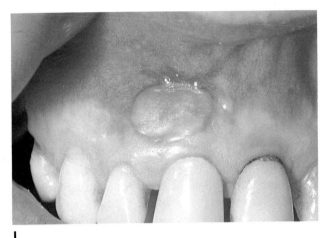

k

l

Figure 17.21 a, Unsightly amalgam tattoo 1⌋ **b,** Tinfoil template trimmed to completely cover the tattoo. **c,** Bevelled incision around the recipient site. **d,** Sharp dissection of affected granulation tissue. **e,** The prepared recipient bed on periosteum and bone. **f,** Marking incision around the tinfoil template on keratinized palatal mucosa. **g,** Undermining incision 1–2 mm deep. **h,** Graft retracted by means of a silk suture and further developed by sharp dissection. **i,** Graft held in place by four 4/0 silk sutures. **j,** Periodontal dressing covering the recipient bed. **k,** Donor site protected by a carboxymethyl cellulose dressing retained by an acrylic stent. **l,** The grafted site 6 weeks postoperatively.

sterile tinfoil so that it completely covers the discoloured area of mucosa, overlapping by a width of 1–2 mm (Figure 17.21b). A shallow incision is then made around the template, extending in depth to just within the connective tissue. The area thus delineated is known as the recipient site. The template is then put aside, being first marked in such a way that the operator knows which is the tissue side.

The recipient site is now prepared by controlled dissection through the marker incision. The angle of the wound edge is bevelled downwards and inwards within the keratinized mucosa (Figure 17.21c) in order to facilitate adaptation of the graft during healing, which will lead to a better postoperative appearance. Deeper connective tissues which are infiltrated by amalgam are thoroughly removed by a process of sharp dissection and curettage (Figure 17.21d). Wherever possible, a connective tissue bed of fibrous tissue or periosteum is preserved intact, especially over root prominences where fenestration or dehiscence of the alveolar bone may occur (Figure 17.21e). However, if unavoidable, a recipient bed of alveolar bone can be accepted.

The donor site

The free mucosal graft donor site can be any area of easily accessible keratinized tissue, and is usually the palatal mucosa in the molar region. An adequate infiltration of anaesthesia will elevate the reflective mucosa slightly, and will improve access and haemostasis. The tinfoil template is placed with the 'tissue' side on the mucosa. In order to avoid cutting the palatal ⌐

blood vessels the superior edge of the tinfoil should be below the maximum point of reflected mucosa.

A marking incision about 3 mm deep is made around the template (Figure 17.21f) and the graft is dissected out through this access wound. Sharp dissection is used, in a plane parallel to the overlying mucosa contour and at a depth of 1–2 mm, thin enough for the operator to see the 'shadow' of the underlying scalpel blade (Figure 17.21g). It is sensible to pass a suture through the mesial part of the detaching mucosa at an early stage of the dissection (Figure 17.21h). Such a manoeuvre will aid the progressive reflection and maintenance of the graft, and will simplify this delicate stage of the operation. It will also prevent the embarrassment of explaining to the patient the loss of a suddenly released, unrestrained graft that he or she has swallowed, or that has been aspirated.

Once the graft has been released, it may, if too thick, be placed on a piece of saline-wettened gauze and the thickness reduced by careful sharp dissection of the connective tissue surface.

An alternative to the tinfoil template technique is the use of a hand or handpiece-driven mucotome. This, however, produces a graft of set width, which may not be appropriate for the site on which it is to be placed.

Placement of graft at recipient site

The graft is now sutured to the fixed margins or connective tissue bed of the recipient site with 4/0 black silk or polyglycolate sutures (Figure 17.21i). The smallest number of sutures sufficient to prevent migration and mobility of the graft needs to be placed.

Gentle pressure is temporarily exerted on the graft with dampened gauze, both to ensure adaptation and eliminate unnecessary dead space. After a few minutes a periodontal pack such as Coe-pack should be placed (Figure 17.21j).

Protection of donor site

The donor site can be particularly painful during healing and should be protected. Coe-pack may be used attached to adjacent teeth, or another dressing such as a carboxymethyl cellulose adhesive may be held in place by means of a clasp-retained acrylic baseplate (Figure 17.21k).

Postoperative care

A chlorhexidine mouthwash should be used for approximately 1 month postoperatively. Dressings and sutures are removed at 7–10 days.

The postoperative appearance of the graft, when seen close-to, seldom exactly matches that of the adjacent mucosa and the patient must be warned of this (Figure 17.21l). However, the contrast is so slight as to be unnoticeable to a casual observer.

Chapter 18

Examination; Treatment Plan; Preoperative Preparation; Prognosis

The previous chapters have dealt with the technical procedures and problems associated with endodontic surgery. It is now possible, on the basis of these facts, to discuss treatment planning.

A preliminary appointment should be made prior to surgery, in order to take a history, make an examination and determine a treatment plan. The need for, and the nature of the operation, should be explained to the patient, as should the likelihood of postoperative sequelae and the prognosis. Preoperative instructions should be given.

Examination and Treatment plan

Once the history and examination have been undertaken it is helpful to make a checklist of eight questions.

(1) Which tooth or teeth require(s) treatment?

(2) Is apicectomy the correct treatment?

(3) What is the morphology of the tooth and the adjacent tissues?

(4) What type of flap should be raised?

(5) What type of seal should be placed?

(6) Are associated structures at risk?

(7) Is the case suitable for treatment in the surgery?

(8) Does the medical history preclude treatment?

Which tooth or teeth require(s) treament?

The tooth to be treated must be positively identified, on the basis of the following investigations.

History

The memory of both the nature and the location of pain is often imprecise. Nevertheless, the history given by the patient will usually direct the examination to the relevant tooth, certainly to the affected area of the jaw. Other recollections may be of value. The occurrence of sudden pain during endodontic treatment may, for example, suggest a root fracture or perforation.

Visual examination

The following signs should be sought:

(1) *Sinuses.* The orifice of a sinus tract may lie at some distance away from the area of pathology from which it arises. The source of the sinus can often be identified by carefully passing a fine gutta-percha point along the tract, confirming its position by means of a radiograph (Figure 18.1)

(2) *Swellings of the mucosa or underlying bone*

(3) *Discolouration of the mucosa.* An amalgam tattoo will often indicate the presence of metallic debris in the tissues above a previously apicected root (Figure 18.2)

(4) *Discoloured teeth*

(5) *Unduly mobile teeth*

(6) *Periodontal pocketing.* The gingival crevice of the suspect tooth should be carefully examined for the presence of pockets, using a fine diagnostic probe. Deep pockets arising as a result of the longstanding drainage of pus from an apical lesion require an envelope flap to be raised so that the contaminated root surfaces may be thoroughly planed and debrided along their whole length. Inaccessible, palatally placed pockets may be the cause of apicectomy failure, and are particularly difficult both to diagnose and treat.

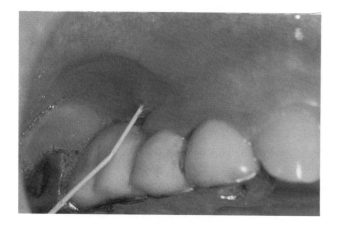

a

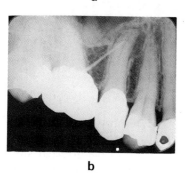

b

Figure 18.1 a, *Gutta-percha point gently passed up a sinus tract.* **b,** *A radiograph confirms the source of the sinus to lie some distance from the orifice. (Different case to that illustrated in Figure 18.1a)*

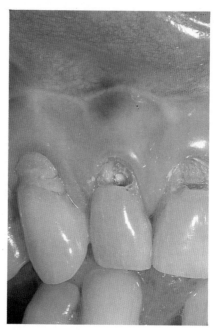

Figure 18.2 *Amalgam tattoo of the mucosa above an apicected 2|*

Radiographic examination

Radiographs must be taken. Because of superimposition, a single radiograph may fail to reveal every root and root canal. Similarly, root fractures, perforations, and lateral canals may not be identified. It is thus sensible routinely to expose two radiographs with the tube placed at different antero-posterior angles. An orthopantomograph is useful for determining the position of the inferior dental canal and mental foramen in those cases where a lower tooth is to be apicected (Figure 18.3).

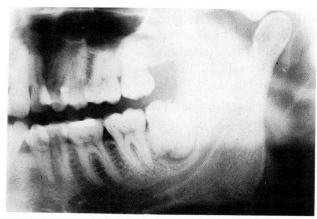

Figure 18.3 *The positions of the inferior dental canal and the mental foramen can usually be seen on an orthopantomograph*

Vitality tests

The (usual) non-vitality of the tooth to be treated must be determined preoperatively, and the vitality or non-vitality of the adjacent teeth must also be checked. Vitality testing is of particular importance when radiographs show the roots of several teeth to be associated with an apical lesion. Electric pulp testers should not be relied upon to determine fine variations in the degree of vitality, but simply whether or not the tooth is vital. It is essential that the tooth under test be electrically insulated from its neighbours, lest false positive responses are recorded. Insulation can be ensured by placing small squares of rubber dam between the mesial and distal contact points (Figure 18.4). The application of heat

and cold may also be used as a diagnostic test. On occasions it is possible to determine vitality only by drilling a small test cavity into the dentine of the unanaesthetized tooth. Pain will usually, though not inevitably, be felt before a vital pulp is exposed.

Is apicectomy the correct treatment?

Once the tooth requiring treatment has been identified, it is necessary to decide whether or not an apicectomy can be justified as being the correct treatment.

For example:

(1) Can the tooth, or one or more of its roots be treated by means of conventional root canal filling techniques?

(2) Can the tooth be restored?

(3) Is the tooth of value in the whole-mouth treatment plan?

(4) Would an alternative form of treatment (i.e. extraction, followed by bridgework) offer a more realistic chance of long-term success?

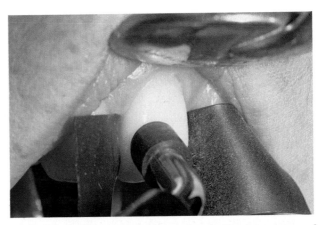

Figure 18.4 *When checking pulp vitality by means of an electric pulp tester, the teeth must be insulated. This may be done by placing rubber dam between the contact points*

What is the morphology of the tooth and the adjacent tissues?

Once apicectomy has been decided upon, a detailed visual and radiographic study must be made of both the tooth and the adjacent tissues. It is important that potential problems are identified prior to operation.

(1) The angulation of the crown and hence the likely position and depth of the roots.

(2) The number and shape of the roots.

(3) The number and conformation of the root canals.

(4) The presence of root fractures and perforations.

(5) The extent and probable nature of any apical pathology.

What type of flap should be raised?

The following factors should be noted and used to determine the design of the muco-periosteal flap that is to be raised.

(1) The presence of inflamed mucosa, sinus tracts and periodontal pockets

(2) The presence of fraena, and the widths of the mucosa and attached gingiva

(3) The presence of artificial crowns and associated gingival recession

(4) The presence of prominent roots and thin mucosa, suggesting underlying dehiscences

As determined radiographically:

(5) The angulation of the tooth root in relation to its crown

(6) The position and size of associated lesions in the alveolar bone

(7) The position of the maxillary antrum

(8) The position of the mental foramen

What type of seal is to be placed?

As far as possible, the operator should decide preoperatively, which obturation technique he intends to use. The decision is made on the basis of the clinical investigation (for example, are the root canals patent?) and the radiographic evidence. The decision may require to be altered in the light of problems encountered during surgery.

Are associated structures at risk?

If there is the slightest risk of involvement, the positions of the mental nerve (foramen), the inferior dental nerve (canal) and maxillary antrum must be positively identified.

Is the case suitable for treatment in the surgery?

Most simple apicectomies may be done under local anaesthesia, on an outpatient basis. However, deeply placed roots, multiple lesions, large cysts, the proximity of the antrum, and the patient's age or ill health may be good reasons to hesitate and consider referring the patient for specialist advice and treatment.

Preoperative Preparation

Control of infection

Only in exceptional circumstances should endodontic surgery be undertaken in the presence of acute apical infection. Infection should first be controlled by the appropriate use of drainage, dressings and antibiotics.

Preparation of the root canals

Roots that are amenable to conventional endodontic treatment, and which are not to be apicected – for example, the palatal root of upper molars – should be instrumented and filled prior to operation. If an ortho-grade seal is to be placed at the time of apicectomy, the access cavity should be prepared preoperatively and the entrances to the root canals identified.

Further preparations

When appropriate, cast gold post and cores should be prepared and temporary restorations constructed. If there is a likelihood that the operation might not successfully be completed (for example, when an at-tempt is to be made to repair a perforation), a denture or, exceptionally, a temporary bridge may be prepared for immediate postoperative placement. When replant-ation is to be done, a soft splint must be prepared.

Preoperative Instructions

Most adult patients appreciate a simple explanation of the principles of root canal therapy and the nature of apicectomy. They will often ask about the advisability of eating immediately preoperatively, and whether they should attend accompanied. The question of sedation may arise. The patient should be apprised of the likeli-hood of postoperative discomfort, swelling and bruis-ing. Many will ask how soon (or delayed) may be their return to work. The prognosis must be discussed.

Prognosis

Patients will often ask for an assessment of prognosis in order to help them decide whether or not to submit to apicectomy. Such advice is not easy to give. Whereas it is usually a simple matter to identify the number and position of the roots and root canals, other factors cannot so easily be determined. For example, how deeply placed is the root-tip? Is there an unidentified root fracture? Will profuse bleeding obscure the root apex or contaminate the seal? At this stage it is probably best to offer the patient a judgement in general terms, such as 'good chance', 'fair chance' and 'worth an attempt'. It should, however, be explained to the patient that it will be possible to give a more positive assessment as soon as the operation has been completed, and a satisfactory seal placed.

Medico-legal

It is good practice to maintain detailed clinical case notes. In the light of the current climate of increasing litigation it is also sensible to explain techniques and problems visually as well as verbally. Explanatory sketches should be made in, or stapled to, the patients' case notes.

Index